It's Going To Be OK

The journey of a mother's five-year wait
to finally have a child

Dear Claire,

*All the best in everything and
God bless.*

Chumi

Chumi Lakshmi Sinnanchetty

malcolm down

PUBLISHING

Copyright ©2022 Chumi Lakshmi Sinnanchetty

First published 2022 by Malcolm Down Publishing Ltd
www.malcolmdown.co.uk

26 25 24 23 22   7 6 5 4 3 2 1

British Library Cataloguing in Publication Data
A catalogue record for this book is available from the British Library.

ISBN 978-1-915046-25-3

Cover design by Laxman Sivanathan
Art direction by Sarah Grace

Printed in the UK

Dedication

To my beautiful, loving son, Levi, not only have you birthed a mother in me, but you have also unleashed a side of me that I never knew existed.

To my husband Laxman, you are the wind beneath my wings. You believed in me even when I didn't.

To my mother, it was you who got the ball rolling.

To those who see but not believe, hear but not listen, everyone who's reading this and everyone who's on a journey to your promise, I know how it feels, but don't give up.

Acknowledgements

No man is an island. As such, there are a few people whom I must thank and express my heartfelt gratitude, not only in writing this book, but for standing by me throughout my shaky journey towards finally receiving the God-given promise.

First and foremost, to my husband. You wouldn't be reading this had it not been for Laxman who never failed to nudge me to achieve my full potential, to the extent that he chased me out of the house (and my comfort zone) one cold Saturday morning in January 2022, so I could sit in Costa and concentrate on getting this book done. Thank you for challenging me to take the leap and for the occasional company at 4am while I was finishing up this book.

To my family, you do not know how much your presence and support has carried me through difficult times in the last six years of my journey. Thank you for standing by my side through thick and thin.

A big token of appreciation also goes to my publisher, Malcolm, for patiently answering my never-ending questions and for bending over backwards to make my vision a reality under such short notice. I still can't believe he agreed.

They are never going to read this, but I must also thank the staff in Costa who graciously allowed me to warm their seat for four hours on busy Saturday mornings with only one hot chocolate.

Contents

Prologue

If there was one question that could win the trophy as the most asked question in my entire married life, it would be, "When is the baby coming?" Had I had an answer to it, I would have every right to claim God's throne as my own. Fortunately, and unfortunately, I never had an answer to that question. For someone who thrives on plans and schedules, knowing exactly what she would eat or wear every week, having to-do lists for everything in her life, and a diary planned to the T, uncertainties that tag along with such questions lead to a disastrous end.

Before Levi, the question was – *When is the baby coming?*

After Levi, the question is now – *What is your story?*

Because I wouldn't shut up about how Levi was a promise from God to me and, contrary to popular belief, it wasn't an answer to a Hannah's prayer.[1] Whenever possible, I never fail to make a statement that Levi is not a result of the pandemic in 2020. Neither was it because I was well rested while working from home. You will understand why as the story unfolds.

Let me give you a bit of a backstory so you can catch up to present time.

I am a Malaysian, with Indian ancestors, living in the UK ever since I moved here to pursue my postgrad degree. I have been married to Laxman since April 2015 and intend to be married to him till death do us part. In April 2021, we were blessed with the sweetest and most loving little boy called Levi.

The six-year gap between my marriage and the birth of Levi sometimes felt like a complete nightmare, only because of the aforementioned reason in the first paragraph of this chapter.

7

When we first found out I was pregnant in August 2020, I would have wanted to publish it on Facebook saying, "Hah, in your face! Now leave me alone," but of course I didn't. I am far too cultured for that.

To be honest, both Laxman and I were shocked ourselves and it took us a good couple of days for it to sink in. One evening in August 2020, I was decluttering my drawers and found a digital pregnancy kit. It was one of those expensive ones that would display the words "Pregnant" or "Not pregnant" and tell you an estimation of how many weeks, too, should it be positive. In all honesty, it's just an over glorified expensive pregnancy test kit, which I clearly fell for. I did not even have the slightest clue that pregnancy test kits could expire. I bought it four years earlier as a backup just for the thrill of seeing the word "Pregnant" rather than a double line or a positive sign. Since it was expensive, I didn't even want to randomly use it without multiple positives from the cheaper ones first. In the end, I never had the chance to use it all those years and it was buried deep in my drawer all along.

By the time I found this unused package in my drawer, I was quite numb internally, so it didn't really bother me that it had been knocking about for so many years and I never had the opportunity to use it. The expiry date printed on the box caught my eye and I realised it had expired a few days ago. I paid some £20 for it and saved it for such a long time. I wasn't going to throw it out unopened now! So, I left it in my bathroom that night to be used first thing in the morning, as testing first thing in the morning would give the most accurate results. Well, it had already expired, I don't know why I still wanted to follow the instructions.

When I woke up on 5th August at 5am, I almost forgot about it until I saw it sitting on the sink waiting for me. Void of all emotions,

I sat there waiting for the words "Not pregnant" to appear so that I could throw it in the bin and carry on with regular programming that Wednesday morning. Two minutes later, I saw the word "Pregnant" and woke up with the jolt. It threw me completely off guard. I rushed out of the toilet to get Laxman who had just woken up and had no clue what I was up to. We both stared at it for the longest time. We dared not rejoice, thinking it might be too soon, and couldn't brush it off because it said "Pregnant"! It wasn't even the right time of the month yet to test.

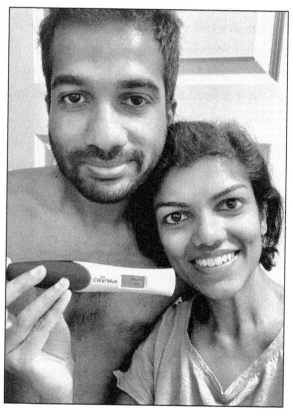

First picture we took when we found out on 5th August 2020.

It was like a double-edged sword. We didn't want to allow unbelief to overtake the joy and, yet, we were too nervous to fully accept it. What if this doesn't stay? What if it was a false positive? It was an expired stick after all. You bet I went out and got multiple cheap pregnancy kits to test the whole week and even multiple times a day.

Eventually, with time, we started relaxing and we knew this baby was here to stay. However, the fact that I was finally pregnant did not heal the wound and the scars that burnt me deep within over the years.

It's very common to not have a child immediately after marriage. It's OK to not understand what God is trying to tell you there and then. There's no need to assume something is wrong with you all the time. Sometimes I wished life was more transparent and people were more open about it instead of always questioning me, which in turn made me question God.

So here I am, writing the book I wish I had when I was searching for answers. This is not the type of book where I talk about my plight and journey or boast about what I have and how it happened. There is absolutely nothing to boast about me. It is not intended to cause any triggers or heartaches for anyone. This is my account of how God sustained me and carved out everything in my life unbeknown to me. It's always about Him.

I am usually an open book, not hesitating to lend my voice about conflicts for the benefit of others and always being real. Regardless, I've carefully guarded this part of my life away from the public eye, including family and friends. It has been tremendously challenging to pry open this highly secretive chapter of my life in this book, because it was shut with double doors, bolted with an iron pin-numbered lock for which I've attempted to forget the password. But in obedience to God, it needed to be done. This book has been a long time in the making, more than five years to be exact.

As I stumble through my words and share my most vulnerable periods of life and thoughts with you, I only have one request of you while you are reading this book. Please do not garner any sympathy or empathy for me when you read my story. I'm one of those odd people who cannot function well with either of them, hence I had decided when I was much younger that I would do absolutely everything I could in my power to never willingly put myself in a situation where I would have to face either of them.

My hope is that you will see God. It's always about Him.

The Promise

∽

Every girl's dream is to get married, have children, and have her own family.

Or so I've heard.

I wasn't one of them though. During our gloriously single and youthful years, most of my friends would talk about how they wanted their wedding day to be and what attributes they wanted in a husband. I would passively listen and not participate or contribute to that discussion. They were all far too excited to even notice my silence whenever this topic came up. I never had any imaginary wedding plans in my childhood, or even adulthood for that matter.

Truth be told, I never wanted to get married, let alone plan to have children. But when marriage talks were finally on the table, the transition from not wanting to get married at all to actually getting married was an interesting one. Since it wasn't something I had anticipated, I only lived in the moment and took one thing at a time. It was too overwhelming to process the sudden change that marriage brought. I didn't have any mental capacity to think of anything else beyond that. The goal was to get married first, then learn to live with someone else and love this person like the Bible tells me to, or at least show some respect and love to begin with. And, of course, stay married to this person.

If marriage was such a long and hard process for me, having children was even more difficult. Therefore, I didn't give it much thought or planning. For a serial planner like me, not having any plans is nearly impossible. The only two things in my life that I didn't plan were my marriage and children. To be fair, I am a strong believer that I could not control these two if I were to give them to God completely, which I did all along. I have always wanted God's plans for me rather than the permissible option that I could possibly have. Therefore, I never even attempted to plan for these.

It might sound as if I resent getting married or being married. It's neither. I peacefully accepted the proposal and marriage. It couldn't have been clearer that it was God's perfect plan for me when it eventually did happen.

At the time of writing this book, I've been married for six years and I have absolutely no regrets. I've known for quite a few years now that this has been the best plan and person that God had for me.

I settled with the man quite easily. But it wasn't easy dealing with the next stage in a married life.

The promise to my mother

Before it was arranged that I would marry Laxman, there were years of gruelling process looking at potential alliances. Because I wasn't yet warmed up to the idea of marriage back then, the process was so tiresome and frustrating to me, to the extent that I never even wanted to talk about it.

It was during this time that my mother shared with me about how God had promised her that He would bless her family and enlarge her tent. I remember her being so emotional when she shared it and the Bible verse that the Holy Spirit had given her to confirm the promise. She went on and on about how it was a promise that God was going to fulfil through me when I got married and had children.

That's the vague description that I remembered of that episode, not really the verses and everything else she said. Very honestly, I wasn't paying much attention. In my defence, firstly, I wasn't interested in marriage. Secondly, it didn't make any sense to me because I didn't even want to get married. How would something about having children be relevant to me when I wasn't enthusiastic about the idea of being married. And finally, the entire hope just didn't appeal to me back then. It was my mother's promise, not mine.

My mother was the one to have fantasies about my wedding for years and years while I was frolicking in the meadows of studies, work and just life in general. Between the two of us, she was definitely the one who would pray about it and wait upon God to reveal the right person and His promises, etc. While I, on the other hand, refused to have anything to do with it.

After years of denial about ever getting married, I thought I wasn't interested in the word that my mother received but, unconsciously, I carried it at the back of my mind all along.

The promise to me

In April 2015, some time after the promise that my mother shared with me, I got married. Five days after we got married in Malaysia, Laxman left to come back to the UK while I stayed back in Malaysia, waiting for my UK spouse visa. It was such a long and tedious process that it took us a good eight months to apply and receive the decision that my application was successful and that I could travel back to the UK in December 2015.

During this eight-month period, I had encountered so many unwarranted questions about expanding our family. Even more so after Laxman's second visit to Malaysia in July 2015. The second visit was a short two-week trip combined as a belated birthday trip for me and for the spouse visa application evidence. You'd be surprised by the number of questions I had after those two weeks.

I was so furious. Why would someone want you to be pregnant while you are all alone? This generation is no longer like older Asian generations where husbands worked overseas throughout the year and could only travel back to their home country to visit their wife and children or to impregnate said wife and then leave almost immediately to go back to work to support the family. No, I'm not from that generation. And I did not get married just for the sake of having children. I wasn't going to be pregnant while I was all alone in Malaysia with no certainty about when I could go back to the UK. I hadn't had a chance to get to know Laxman properly or even live a proper married life. I wasn't even sure if I was wife material, how would I be ready to be mother material?

Amid all these offensively invasive questions and my own frustration, I heard God loud and clear. I've had several experiences in the past where God has spoken to me when I was like young Samuel, unaware that it was God calling me or speaking to me. But that was many moons ago. By August 2015 though, my conversations with God had become more of a two-way communication. I was rather seasoned with God's ways and voice in my life.

One fine August morning in 2015 while I was pottering about in my house, God spoke to me. I hadn't initiated a conversation, nor was I even actively seeking to hear from Him. He spoke about the Abrahamic covenant and told me that it was His promise to me about my family. First, He said that He would make me into a great nation,[2] and then He added on to say that He would make my offspring like the dust of the earth.³ That's all. Those words shook me from my mundane morning. There was so much to unpack from those words. How do I unpack them? What do I do with this promise that I didn't actively seek? Make me into a great nation? Make my offspring like the dust of the earth? Do you know how much dust there actually is on the face of the earth? How am I going to handle such a huge responsibility? I didn't ask for any of this. I didn't ask to be a great nation. I cannot handle any attention in a small congregation, let alone a nation!

Needless to say, I was confused for quite some time. I spent a lot of time reading the Bible, trying to understand the Abrahamic covenant. I hadn't understood everything, I don't think I even fully believed what I heard from God for a good couple of months. Nonetheless, it was a promise that I held close to my heart. What I wasn't aware of at that time was that it would be something that would prolong for years to come. My mother's words from years ago came flooding back, but because I didn't pay too much attention to her back then, I just added it like a piece to the puzzle. It was an incomplete puzzle for a very long time.

It could have been that I was in disbelief myself for some time that I didn't speak about this promise to anyone. Not even to Laxman or my mother. I let it rest on the back burner while I carried on with life. Maybe it was a mistake. I don't think I heard it right. It would have been for someone else. So many *maybe, could have,* and *would have* scenarios kept playing in my head in relation to the promise.

The promise to Laxman

In October 2015, my spouse visa was approved, allowing me to travel to the UK in December 2015. December 2015 had finally come and off I was to the UK to be reunited with my husband in Bristol. The excitement of relocating and settling into my new life was so great that I no longer paid much attention to the promise.

During Christmas 2015, Laxman and I visited my church in Glasgow and the visiting speaker, who hadn't met me or Laxman before and didn't know of our history, looked Laxman dead in the eye and prophesied the Abrahamic covenant over him, the exact same words that God had spoken to me four months before. It wasn't even like a prayer for Laxman, but the exact words that God had told me. Laxman was unphased; I was the opposite! But I held my poker face that night.

That was the third time! *I wonder if God is trying to tell me something.*

Once the Christmas season was over and we were all back to our regular routine in Bristol in the new year, I cautiously started talking about it to Laxman. I shared about the promise with him, and we both discussed it.

It sounds as if we sat at a board meeting talking about the promise and laying out our plans to see how they aligned with the promise. No, we didn't. I had finally opened up about it to Laxman after almost half a year of me hearing it.

Given the nature of our marriage where circumstances led me to move back to Malaysia right after the engagement, we didn't even have the opportunity to think about what our goals in life were, how many children we wanted, and other basic things a lot of couples usually plan before they get married. All we knew when we decided we were going to marry was that God had ordained us to be together, so we were getting married. Only after moving in together in December 2015 did it sink in that we were now married. So, it made more sense to speak about children then, but neither of us could really comprehend the Abrahamic covenant in our lives.

What would you do if it were you who'd had all these promises and confirmations?

What was I supposed to do with such a promise? I did not have a clue what I was to do with it. It was far greater than I could comprehend, and it came at a time when I hadn't the slightest desire or plans for children. But that doesn't mean I didn't want any children. I hadn't mentally prepared for it, hence why I felt I needed more time.

I just wasn't the type who lived in a fantasy world thinking about how many children I would have and what their names would be, and how my morning routine and night routine would be when sending kids to school or dressing them up for a family photoshoot.

Also, all my life, I grew up with minimal or absolutely no attention from anyone drawn towards me. I was happy to be a wallflower. Abrahamic covenant is no joke. When something so big was suddenly promised to me, I didn't think I could handle it.

The Process

Imagine this:

You are watching an extremely interesting nail-biting movie with someone else, say Avengers: Endgame *from Marvel. Your movie partner pauses the movie just when you are on the edge of your seat waiting for the climax. What's going to happen to Thanos? What will happen to Iron Man if he snaps his fingers? Will he survive? What even is Avengers without Iron Man? (Apologies to any non-Marvel fans who do not get this reference. It's OK, you haven't missed much. And this will be the only Marvel reference in this whole book.)*

Your movie partner needs to attend to some other business. More important than Endgame *apparently. He proceeds to leave the room without any warning as to why he is going out, how long he will be out or when he will return. Most importantly, he leaves with the remote.*

It's one of those futuristic television screens where there are no manual controls. You are now stuck because you cannot watch the movie to see what happens next. You are even more frustrated because you don't know when he's coming back because he hadn't mentioned anything. Above all else, you are just plain annoyed because there is no closure, and you can't get it out of your head.

What could be more important than finishing the movie? Your only choice is between waiting or forgetting about the movie.

How would you feel if I were to tell you to add five years to the waiting game?

Yup, that's exactly how I felt.

For many years I was furious with God because He had pressed pause in my life. I searched for the remote high and low, and tried to make things move in my own might, so that I could take control of it once again. On days when I was extremely frustrated with the lack of clarity, the Holy Spirit would gently remind me that I had proactively decided that I was going to allow God to have supremacy in my life over my own desires and plans. I would always suffix my prayers with "Let your will be done, God".

Be careful what you pray for, they say.

I have absolutely no regrets asking God to take control. But I was reluctant to let Him have full control over the baby department. I just couldn't tolerate not knowing what was going to happen next and when.

If there's only one thing you should know about me, or rather one thing that's very obvious, it's my impatience. I have no patience whatsoever. If I want something, I need it instantly. Which explains why I am fan of big giants like Amazon; purely for the benefit of their Prime next-day delivery. Such is my impatience. I'm not proud of it, neither do I make any attempts to overcome it. It's a harmless attitude to want to be organised and stay on top of everything as much as I can, which is usually nine times out of ten. It is, after all, some harmless shopping website. I have no regrets about it and I make no apologies for it. But this impatience has clearly spilled through many other areas in my life, the baby being one of them.

GP

Laxman and I started our fertility investigative journey around autumn 2016. It had been more than half a year since I moved to the UK and we had already missed several pregnancies by then. With everyone's wellbeing in mind, I shall not be going into details of the missed pregnancies or of the investigations. We thought there were some complications, so we went to our GP. Looking back now at the way things panned out ever since we decided we were going to go through the investigation route, I realise we were so naïve. We were not aware of how long the investigations would take and how emotionally consuming this was going to be. It felt like walking blindfolded in a jungle full of thorny creepers, if I'm honest, but it had to be done. I was consumed by the thought that something could be wrong and that I needed to do something to fix it.

Fertility investigations always start with the woman first, and almost nothing for the man until almost the last stages of investigation. It's very lopsided but I'm not about to begin a rant about how unfair that seems. My GP started off by asking me a whole bunch of questions about my family history and told me that I had to do a set of blood tests to begin with. GP surgeries were only open during working hours and blood tests needed to be done first thing in the morning so the samples could be sent to the lab on time. Since I couldn't go to my local GP, we had to book an appointment for me to go to a partner GP practice which was open much earlier so that I could drop in before work. The earliest appointment was three months later. One cold morning in December 2016, I went to the appointed GP practice to have my bloods done. They told me that it could take several weeks and that my own GP would contact me once the results were available. I waited till after the whole Christmas and New Year holidays were over. Blood works usually need to be processed and tested within a day or two, or else they will no longer yield any reliable results. But over Christmas and New Year holidays, it somehow becomes OK to wait for weeks.

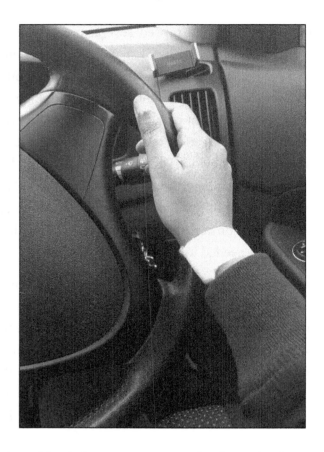

I hadn't heard back from my GP even by the end of January 2017, so I contacted them, only to be told that my blood tests hadn't been done at all. It took several phone calls between both the GP practices and the labs to figure out that the second GP practice had not even sent my bloods to the lab, or that the lab had misplaced the samples. The bottom line was that someone had lost all the tubes of blood that they took from me, and no one was owning up to it. I needed to get another test done. A few more months went past before this was done. The GP didn't find anything wrong with my bloods and referred me to a fertility centre nearby.

Fertility clinic 1

The closest fertility centre to me back then was thirty miles away from me, and was only open during working hours, which meant another speed bump in our journey. Both Laxman and I had to take the day off from work to make it to this appointment, and since the NHS is always busy, it took another couple of months before we managed to book an appointment. I walked in to my first appointment in the fertility clinic thinking I was going to be speaking with a consultant, but it was the consultant's nurse instead. She asked me the same set of questions that my own GP had asked almost a year ago, forcing me to recall all the missed pregnancies. She then ordered a couple more blood tests in addition to the ones I had already done. They couldn't do it in the hospital, so I had to go back to my own GP to get it done. She gave me their hospital labelled test tubes and pouches with the correct codes so that my blood tests wouldn't be lost or misplaced.

Guess what? They most definitely were lost. And again, no one was willing to take any responsibility. My GP said they never received the results from the lab; the lab said the bloods never reached them.

The hospital offered me another appointment to do the blood tests a few months down the road. How was it that they couldn't do it the first time round, but suddenly able to the second time? This was already June 2017. My frustration with the system and services led me to decline their offer. I truly appreciate the work of the NHS but sensitive cases like fertility investigations should be handled with more care and not just as another case with some random codes on a piece of paper.

I didn't think doing another blood test with the hospital this time was going to help us much or fast track anything. It took a year and a half to do a few blood tests, talk about our experiences multiple times and never really get anywhere. We were swamped with work and buying a house during that period anyway. It was a good distraction that I created for myself. We decided to park it temporarily and focus on our house purchase and move. I kept myself so busy with the house and my work that I hardly had any time to think about it. It is so much easier on the heart and mind when there's something else to focus on.

Fertility clinic 2

Following our move in September 2017, we delayed registering at the new GP in our local area until January 2018. We both agreed that it was about time to resume the process from where we had left it. What we thought was resuming, ended as starting fresh on a clean slate because it was a new GP and they had absolutely no clue about our history. Why do they make a note of everything on their computers during each appointment? And what takes them so long for the health board to transfer medical notes from one GP to another if there aren't many notes?

That was the third time I spoke to a GP about my history. We went through the whole lot of questions all over again, recalling each date and experience. We were then referred to another fertility clinic (which will be referred to as fertility clinic 2 from here onwards) local to us, which was about five miles away. The referral took about three months due to some sort of miscommunication. My GP told me they would write to fertility clinic 2, who would then contact me. They didn't, so I chased them up and was told that they never received any referral. So, I had to go back to my GP who promised to send another referral, which they did online this time. I'm guessing it was a new system because fertility clinic 2 had received it, but overlooked it.

Meaning it was sitting in the equivalent of their junk mailbox until I called and chased them up.

By the time we got to see someone at fertility clinic 2, my blood tests had expired. So, the consultant requested a new set of blood tests. She scribbled the names of the tests that needed to be done on an envelope that she could get hold of from her desk and passed it to me along with some test tubes and pouches with bar codes that would allow the correct scanning process in the labs.

For some wild reasons unknown to me, consultants or other departments always send you to your own GP for blood tests instead of doing it themselves, although they have the facilities to do so. I didn't have a very good feeling about it, but I made an appointment with my GP to get the bloods done, and when I went in for the appointment, the nurse took one quick look at the note from the consultant and refused to do the tests. She didn't know what half of them were (obviously because she didn't work in the fertility department) and refused to accept a handwritten note from someone she didn't know.

Next was obviously another call to my consultant and a couple of days wait for her to return my call. The consultant then sent me a type-written letter under her letter head and said she'd leave notes on my online NHS portal so everyone who has access to my files could see them. Once this was done, I called my GP to make another appointment. The nurse who booked me in said she could see the requests online and that I didn't need to bring the test tubes and pouches with the codes that my consultant had given me.

I shouldn't have listened to her, but I stupidly did. I walked into my blood test appointment the following week before work without those test tubes and pouches, and the nurse who saw me that morning said she couldn't do the tests because they didn't have the appropriate test tubes and pouches for the blood tests that I required.

What a waste of an appointment, time off from work and all the weeks and months I'd spent going back and forth till that date. I came out in tears and frustration that I could no longer contain it. Why would one person tell me one thing over the phone and another person tell me something else? I was losing so much time because of this. I had to take time off from work each time to attend these appointments in the morning and make up for it later in the day. Taking time off from work also meant having to disclose very personal information to my manager, which I wasn't ready to do, and was absolutely not willing to talk about it to my colleagues.

I wanted to give up on the whole investigation and just deal with life as it was. But I had already spent more than two years of my life obsessing over this issue and dodging spears from people who were unapologetically curious about my fertility. I felt the need to have some closure as to why I couldn't get pregnant when Laxman and I didn't have any obvious health issues. I decided to make a third appointment with my GP to do the blood tests requested by my consultant from fertility clinic 2. This time I wasn't taking any more chances, so I took everything I possibly had regardless of what the nurse told me. She took the bloods and said she would drop them off for the lab collection that afternoon; the results would be ready in about a week and would be sent to my consultant at fertility clinic 2, who would then contact me. As if she doubted that I couldn't understand that I shouldn't call her back for the results, she pointed out to me that they would not have access to the results and only my consultant's clinic would. They didn't want me to waste their time by calling them. I knew the consultant wouldn't call me back immediately. So, I gave it about a month and then called my consultant to check if she was going to book me in for another consultation since the bloods were done and she should have had the results.

Surprise! No results were sent to her!

Who do you think now had the job of tracing everything again? Me.

The first call was obviously to my GP. The receptionist at the GP practice said she could see that the bloods were sent off to the lab the afternoon the samples were taken from me but said they couldn't help me any further because the codes meant the results were to be referred to fertility clinic 2; they no longer had any access to the information once the blood samples had been handed to the lab. They wouldn't give me the contact telephone number for the lab or else I would have called them myself. I kind of guilt tripped the receptionist to call the lab for me. Well, they owed me at least that after all the yo-yoing they did with me. The lab denied ever receiving my bloods. How could that possibly happen? Where did they go then? Nobody knows.

Another call to my consultant, and I refused to go back to my GP for more bloods. This time the consultant agreed to get her nurse to take the samples and send the bloods to the lab so the results would come back to them directly. Like the first fertility hospital, fertility clinic 2 also had the capacity to do it themselves from the very beginning, why couldn't they just do it in the first place instead of sending me back to my GP? I guess I will never know the answer to that. Another day, another appointment. Another month or so lost. At least this time they had all the results.

Four appointments and three months later, they found nothing wrong with my bloods. Everything was fine and there was nothing to suggest infertility. The consultant then did a few ultrasound scans in her clinic and suggested that it would be best to have a hysteroscopy and laparoscopy done, which can only be done in the hospital under general anaesthetic.

Hysteroscopy and laparoscopy

I was a tomboy when I was younger, very active in sports and loved running around a lot. I've injured myself many times throughout my lifetime: hurt my shins tripping while running, fractured my wrist when I slipped and fell on soapy water, split open my knees multiple times while playing tennis, sprained my ankles playing softball. I still have most scars to tell the tale, but I have never gone under the knife, nor have I had a general anaesthetic before. This was a whole new level of fear. To be fair, it's in fact a fairly simple procedure with its own set of risks like any other surgery but having not done anything like that before worried me because I didn't know what to expect.

These procedures that I was having done were to check the uterus lining, to ensure there was no endometriosis or anything else. One of my scans had shown potential thickening of the uterus lining, but that could have been due to the time of the month and my consultant wasn't sure, hence the request for a hysteroscopy and laparoscopy to be done to give a definite answer.

Before I could undergo the procedure, I had to have another blood test just to make sure I was healthy enough to have the operation and that there wouldn't be any other complications. They found out that my iron levels were far too low for a surgery with general anaesthetic, so I had to have a blood transfusion done a week before. Another first for the books.

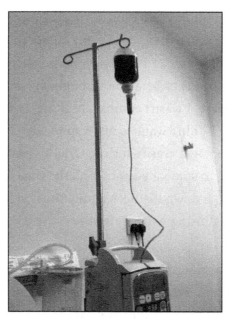

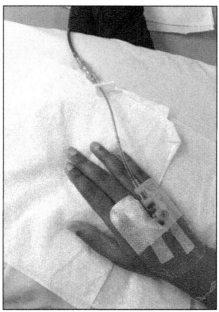

First time getting a blood transfusion before first surgery.

Leading up to the surgery and even during the recovery period, I was so careful not to give anything away to my family and friends. If I were to be honest with myself, I didn't have to be alone throughout the journey. No one needs to be alone throughout such an emotionally draining experience. I wasn't completely alone. Laxman was present at each step, but I didn't want to allow anybody else into it. I knew a huge support system wasn't for me. I didn't want to be whining and complaining to someone about it all the time, and I didn't want someone breathing down my neck all the time asking me how I was doing and sympathising with me just because it's not been an easy journey.

It was a day surgery, so I wasn't required to stay in the hospital, but it took the entire day from signing in to signing out. I took a week off work to recover because I didn't want to go in to work with a bloat and a backache that required me to use a hot pack to nurse it better, along with some rest.

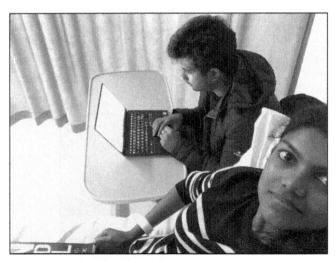

Laxman working away while I was waiting to be wheeled in for surgery

The surgery was done in November 2018, and results were ready the following month. Everything came back as normal. The uterus lining was slightly thickened but that didn't suggest any complications. My consultant didn't find anything wrong with them, indicating nothing was wrong with me. As much as I was relieved that the results had come back normal, I was also frustrated that there wasn't anything wrong that could be treated.

Where do I go from here?

Letrozole

Next step was to encourage ovulation. I had already done multiple blood tests at different times of the month in the past to ensure I was ovulating. Despite this, my consultant suggested pills to encourage ovulation. The pills were called Letrozole, the least invasive method to start off with, and it was only recommended for a month. It was only one tiny little pill that I had to take once a day for three days.

Yeah, sure, I can do that. It's just popping three tiny little pills that won't have much side effect other than slight nausea and potentially twin pregnancies.

I took these pills in January 2019. Two weeks later, I had another scan to check if the pills did what they were supposed to – which was to ensure I was ovulating. They did more than that. Since I was already producing healthy eggs even before the pills, I had produced two eggs that month and the consultant mentioned that there could be a risk of twin pregnancies. To Laxman and me, that was like music to our ears. What risk could there be? We had been struggling this long to have a baby, I was more than happy to take two if I could!

If only conceiving was that easy. Well, it is for a lot of people. Sadly, I wasn't one of them.

Nope, I did not get pregnant that month. What's next?

Hysteroscopy round 2

Since there wasn't anything wrong with either of us, my consultant wasn't able to explain what caused the infertility. Well, she never even mentioned infertility. I wasn't infertile, and so the consultant wasn't able to explain anything. Our final option was to do IVF.

We could choose to do it privately or apply for funding from the NHS. Depending on household income, the NHS would fund the first cycle of IVF treatment. My consultant was going to apply for the NHS funding, but it would be a good couple of weeks before we would receive a response (which meant months). She was confident we would get the funding, so while waiting for the paperwork to be processed, my consultant did another scan and suggested that it would be best to do another hysteroscopy to ensure the uterus lining was all cleaned up again to provide the optimum environment for implantation following IVF.

The second hysteroscopy was done in June 2019. I took another week off work to recover and even went on our annual holiday to Spain after visiting our family in Glasgow. I really needed a break from all that mental and emotional pressure of waiting and not seeing any light at the end of the tunnel. I was more at ease with the second hysteroscopy since I already knew how it would be during the procedure and how I would feel after it. I felt recovery was slightly easier, but I was rather weary of it. I didn't want this to become a pattern. In fact, the second procedure made me even more nervous for IVF. Is this a sign of what is to come in the future? More hospital appointments, more time off work, more hiding and carefully placing my words and tracing my stories when talking to family and friends and even colleagues. I knew I wasn't prepared to share it with anyone, but was I prepared for what was to come, despite not knowing what it was going to be?

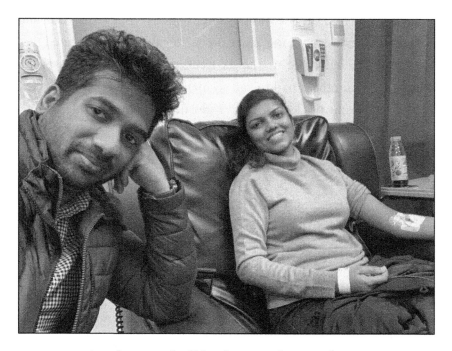

Another round of blood tests and a transfusion.

The concerns I mention about taking time off work was not because my employer wouldn't give it to me. I've had a very understanding manager and employer and I was given all the time off I needed; some of it had to be made up and some of it didn't. Time off work meant I wasn't in the office and my colleagues would notice my absence. My team was a friendly one, they knew a lot about each other. I, on the other hand, was maintaining a very private life regarding this matter. I wanted to avoid giving space for any questions.

What about IVF?

While I was recovering from the second procedure and having a bit of time off to take my mind off this, my consultant had applied for the NHS funding for IVF. She was positive about us being successful, and we were rather hopeful, too, since our medical history indicated that we would be eligible for it. The six-week wait for the NHS response turned into months. I had to call so many departments to get to the bottom of it and track down the right department who dealt with it. Since I was a foreigner under a spouse visa in the UK at the time of applying for the funding, our application was sent to a highly specialised department that did not have any direct contact details.

I remember tagging along with Laxman to Coventry in September 2019 on his work trip so I could take a break but spent all my time calling one department after another to track this down. Having to explain and repeat myself to each department was rather embarrassing. I was sat in a local café to use their Wi-Fi and had to turn away from awkward stares by others. I remember having to control my frustration and tears because I was in a public place and didn't want to cause a scene.

A letter from the NHS finally arrived five months later, stating that I wouldn't be eligible for funding because I was not a permanent resident in the UK back then. I was under a spouse visa, which meant I was paying for NHS treatments.

This carried good news and bad news. The good news was that fertility clinic 2 did both private and NHS IVF treatments in the same building. And if we opted for private treatment, which was the only option left for us now, we would have been able to start it immediately as opposed to having to wait for NHS funding for several more weeks at least, if not months. The bad news was that it would cost about £7,500 and we didn't have the funds. We would have had to either sell my wedding jewellery or take a loan. The latter was more practical, but we both weren't too convinced that it was the wisest decision.

I've heard many times people say having children is expensive, but it really isn't. It's not the babies who have such high demands, it's the parents who choose to spend so much money. If we were going to spend that much money for the IVF to start off with, how would we manage raising the child later? We didn't want to be in debt just for the process and not have enough to spend for when the baby was born.

We had to take a step back and go back to the drawing board – our prayer room (my war room). Waiting for all the procedures and response from the NHS had already taken us into November 2019.

Three years since we first approached our doctor, and we were still nowhere near any sort of solution. It was an extremely painful couple of weeks as we both took some time to pray on our own and seek God for wisdom. On one hand, it looked like IVF was our only option; on the other hand I was questioning God about His promises to me.

After a lot of going back and forth between the three of us – God, Laxman and I – we decided we were going to try and find out more about IVF. Despite me being terrified of the entire process and Laxman sitting on the fence about it, we knew we needed to find out more.

IVF has become so common now that there are many private clinics who offer these services. The only difference is the quality of the service, success rate and the cost. After a lot of searching, we came across a company that had several different methods and one of them was the simplest method for couples with no medical complications. This would only cost us £2,500. I called them in December 2019 and went through so many questions, literally every single step and hypothetical question I could think of. It was the most suitable for us as we met all their criteria, and they had a branch in Bristol too.

They had several appointments for December that they could fit us in, but we didn't want to do it before Christmas because we were going back to Glasgow to be with our family. We couldn't do it right after the New Year because our family was coming back to Bristol to be with us. It was just best not to allow more unwarranted opinions on something so personal and emotional. Laxman and I were a team and we knew we were both sufficient to support each other.

We booked an appointment for February 2020 because that was the best time to start the process. Come February, I chickened out. I decided to postpone it till June that year just before my birthday so that I would still meet their age requirement. We'd been in complete lockdown since March 2020 and, as June was approaching, I was becoming more anxious about it. It could have been because of the delays due to the pandemic; it could have been because I was still terrified of the process. Somehow, I did more digging about the procedures and found out that my understanding about their age requirement was incorrect and that I had more time. We gladly decided to postpone it for another year.

The minute we came to an easy mutual decision on this, both Laxman and I were at complete peace.

We didn't need to rebook an appointment for the following year. We found out I was pregnant in August 2020 when I was checking with an expired pregnancy kit.

After thoughts

So far, it may sound like Laxman didn't have much of a contribution in all this decision making. Trust me when I say we decided on everything together. Since IVF would take more of a toll on me than him, Laxman was gracious enough to allow me to have the final say throughout the process ever since we began our investigative journey in autumn 2016. In fact, it was me who insisted we take the route that we did, and he was supportive all the way through.

Now that I'm writing all this down, I can't help but notice that there was always a delay at every turning point. Sometimes, during the entire journey, I've even wondered whether it was just unfortunate or God's timing that my blood tests and appointments kept getting lost or cancelled. I don't know. It happened EVERY SINGLE TIME, and I was rather oblivious to it back then.

Every time I was sitting in the waiting room, waiting for a doctor's appointment, a blood test or a consultant, I would be lost in my thoughts, sometimes imagining a miracle, that they would find out I was pregnant while doing a scan or a blood test. As months and years passed, those thoughts took a turn for the worse.

I've never been able to accept any sympathy or even empathy for that matter. To me it all sounded and felt the same. While I didn't want it from anyone else, I couldn't help but feel sorry for myself. I hated that feeling. I know hate is a strong word, but that's how it felt then.

Each appointment drained me and robbed me of my joy bit by bit.

The Plague

In layman's terms, the word 'plague' is usually used in reference to something that sticks on to you like a glue and won't budge. Often, it's something bad. In fact, you are doomed if you are hit by a plague. The Book of Exodus talks about the plagues when God was guiding Moses to lead the Israelites out of Egypt.[4] Pharaoh was so hard-hearted that the ten plagues were so extreme.

According to the World Health Organisation (WHO), plague is an infectious disease caused by a bacterium called *Yersinia pestis,* usually found in small mammals and their fleas. It is usually transmitted between animals via their fleas but can also be transmitted from animals to humans via bite, direct contact, or inhalation. Plague is considered a very serious disease in people and can cause 30 per cent to 100 per cent fatality ratio if left untreated. In the fourteenth century, when the plague was first discovered, science wasn't as advanced as it is now. There wasn't enough treatment to contain the severity of the plagues. However, over the years, early diagnosis led to early treatment, which in turn helped curb the intensity of the disease. Despite it sounding very serious, early diagnosis and treatment reduces the risk of fatality.[5]

Such was the state of my mind for a good couple of years – like in the fourteenth century. All I could ever think about was my fertility/infertility journey. I was going crazy thinking about it day and night. It didn't even occur to me that there could be a cure, not just a physical one but a mental and spiritual one too.

Since getting married in April 2015, the questions had already come flooding in, despite Laxman and I living halfway across the world from each other for the first eight months. I always found those questions extremely annoying and difficult to deal with. While I had these questions to deal with, I also had the promise from God that was running at the back of my mind. How do I answer a question that I do not know the answer to, but have an inclination that it would happen? As years passed, I started avoiding meeting family and friends to save myself from answering those questions. If it was completely unavoidable, my answer to such questions changed year after year.

The first year – Smile and politely avoid answering.

The second year – "The baby will come when the time is right."

The third year – "If you are praying about it like you tell me you are, ask God, not me."

The fourth year – "You will know when it happens."

The fifth year – Thank God for the pandemic! (Sounds bad when written, but it was only because I didn't need to face people and face these questions.)

Over time the inclination drifted more towards doubt rather than impatience. I'm hardly ever patient with anything to begin with. So, waiting for something that I thought was a promise obviously started plaguing my mind as a doubt in many ways, shapes and forms.

December 2017 – The start of my negotiations with God

In December 2017, my family from Glasgow came to visit us in Bristol. During the Sunday service, we occupied a whole row in church and I was sat at the end of the row. My first niece, who was two years old back then, jumped from one lap to another till she reached me and wanted to sit with me. If I'm sat down, she would usually go to

Laxman so he could carry her standing up. But that day, she insisted on sitting with me throughout the service and happily playing with my fingers during the sermon. It made me feel warm and fuzzy on the inside – a different kind of love – and triggered the baby fever in me. If you remember from the previous chapter, we had paused our investigations at the fertility clinic during this period when in the midst of waiting for more blood tests from the fertility clinic.

I struck up a deal with God that day. I told God I wanted to be sitting with my own baby this time next year. I was very clear with my request and didn't leave any room for potential mistakes. It's always good to be clear and leave no room for any doubts or loopholes. I wanted to be carrying my baby physically and not just be pregnant. Twelve months is good enough time for that. If He held on to His part of the deal, I would hold on to my part of the deal, which was to stop questioning Him or bothering Him about it ever again. It wasn't so much of a deal at all really, but at that time it sounded fair enough to me.

Come January and February, I was eagerly looking forward to checking if I was pregnant. When March and April rolled around, I changed my deal with God. This time I said that it was OK if I wasn't carrying my baby by December 2018. As long as I was pregnant, I'd be happy. May and June had come and gone with no significant change. I started negotiating again.

My negotiation moved stages very swiftly. It went from being very specific to being lenient, to begging, to threatening that I would stop coming to Him for everything, and finally to fighting. I once told God I would stop talking to Him if He hadn't answered me for this one specific request. I didn't get what I had asked for, but I could never stop talking to Him in the form of fighting. It always ended with,

"Why do you do this to me? Why do you allow me to be humiliated in front of everyone else?"

That's how I felt. Every time someone questioned my fertility, I felt even smaller. It's funny how no one asked Laxman those questions, only to me. Whoever was questioning, it was always directly to me, especially so when I was caught alone without Laxman by my side. Even if Laxman didn't get it from others, he felt the burn from me though, because I couldn't carry it myself.

With every passing month, my communications with God were nothing but bargaining and eventually begging. It didn't quite help that we were being sent back and forth multiple times with lost blood samples and delayed appointments throughout that year too. Come the end of the year, I obviously didn't get what I wanted, neither did I get what God had promised.

The doubt began to creep in. Did I even hear God correctly in the first place? It could have been my imagination, wanting something dramatic to happen. It's not even anything like me to want something flashy that directs attention to me.

Christmas in December 2018 wasn't anything like I had pictured at all. More dreaded questions started flooding in.

April 2018 – Prophecies and prayer training

I gave a reason to myself to be angry with God for everything at any given opportunity. I would always long for some signs and some more confirmation. I hadn't heard from God about His promise since December 2015. The doubt was eating me away. I was sharpening my ears to hear something from God specifically for myself during any sermon or guest speaker's visit or even during any prayer meetings.

I would long for a specific prophecy or direct word from God. If someone else received a prophecy and I didn't, I would be at war with God at home that night.

There was once when I attended a training meeting for leaders who were stepping up to pray for others. It was about submitting ourselves to God and allowing the Holy Spirit to work through us. Throughout the day, there were various activities and several different groups praying for each other and practising. In one of those groups, the lead pastor who was training us walked up to Laxman and prophesied to him. It was a confirmation about his career and studies, nothing to do with the baby. But I was right there next to him, and there was no word for me. Why didn't God speak to me again? Didn't I specifically tell Him that morning that I wanted to hear from Him that day? Why would God no longer speak to me about this despite my numerous attempts at trying to get His attention?

It must have shown that I was miserable on the inside, because the pastor's wife walked up to me at the end of the day asking if I was OK and how I'd found the training. I am the one who hates sympathy and empathy, aren't I? I smiled politely and said everything was good and we had eye-opening training that day. The only thing that was eye-opening to me by the end of the day was that I might have heard it wrong all along.

October 2018 – What about me, God?

One night after Alpha in church, Laxman and I were offering a lift to one of the guests who was a fairly new church member. During conversation on the drive back, she mentioned she couldn't concentrate much on her work or studies because she was always tired and exhausted. I was genuinely concerned about her health, but she casually mentioned it was only because she was eight-weeks pregnant.

Thank God it was Laxman who was driving and I was sat in the front passenger's seat, while the girl was sat at the back. It saved her from seeing the shock I had on my face, and probably a potential jerk had it been me who was driving. She was unmarried and very young. She wasn't even expecting to be pregnant, but of course she embraced the baby and the pregnancy when she found out, despite her partner walking out on her.

What about me, God? Why is it that you would allow this to happen? What am I supposed to learn from this? Why was it that others who were not longing for a baby could get pregnant easily, but me who was having a prolonged medical investigation with no known complications couldn't get pregnant at all?

Receiving pregnancy news from other family members was not one of my favourite things for a long time. When someone announced their pregnancy, the elders would pipe up to say they were waiting for the news from us. Do you know how difficult it has been for me to play it cool? Controlling the tears and watching my facial expressions was the worst of all, especially if it was a Facetime call or in-person meeting.

One Saturday afternoon, Laxman and I went out to the local mall for a stroll and to get some desserts. We were on a low-sugar diet at that time, so we were going to get the smallest dessert and split it between us. Just as we were stood at the counter waiting to place an order, we received a text announcing a fairly close relative was pregnant with their first child after six months of being married. My heart sank. When I reached the counter, I ordered the biggest waffle they had with multiple scoops of ice cream and topped with large bits of Kinder Bueno chocolate pieces. When my dessert arrived, I sat with Laxman and cried my heart out while stuffing my face with the waffle and ice cream. That was one of my coping mechanisms. I would either fight with God or overeat to suppress my emotions. Yes, people were staring at me that day, but nothing bothered me anymore. Worrying about a stranger's perception was the least of my concerns when I felt insignificant in God's eyes. The following week, there was another pregnancy announcement in the family: my in-laws were expecting their third baby.

Each pregnancy announcement sounded to me as if they were mocking me. As time passed, instead of asking me when it was going to be my turn, people would demand that I give them the good news soon.

What about me? Is it too difficult for God to give me one while He can give multiple to others?

Before you jump to any conclusions, I'm happy for everyone who has had their children. Their families are growing, their tents are enlarging. But what about me? Surely God can bless everyone at the same time? Surely God isn't limited with His powers that He can only bless some people and not me. Then why is it that He seems to be doing just that, enlarging others' tents and not mine? I don't care if others are pregnant, why can't I have a child too? Didn't God tell Adam to be fruitful and multiply? Didn't God bless Eve? Why couldn't He do the same for me?

January 2019 – Feeling sorry for myself

The thing about not wanting any attention on myself and not allowing anyone to express any empathy is that I ended up feeling sorry for myself. Since I wouldn't allow it from anyone else, I ended up sympathising with myself. I would continuously look at myself with perspective of a victim. Every time someone asked me how I was doing and was genuinely concerned about our family, my defensive antennas would fling up. I just didn't know how else to respond to people. If I couldn't control myself, I would roll my eyes and say, "It will happen when it happens".

When I could muster up some self-control, I would avoid the topic. I was alert during any conversations. And I avoided meeting well-intended family members at any given chance. Even if someone didn't ask me anything directly, I would treat myself as the victim for being cornered.

Outside my house, I would be smiling and energetic. But inside my four walls, I was as miserable as anyone could ever imagine. Any given chance, I would fight with God. Every single time someone asked me something about not having a baby yet, I would smile on the outside while making an appointment with God to meet in the boxing ring that night. God would be my punch bag at the end of the day. My frustrations had no outlet other than in that boxing ring. My prayers were no longer asking or waiting, they were all of frustrations and accusations.

The funny thing is, despite hitting rock bottom within me and fighting with God about this one particular issue, I was still serving in church. I was still committed to everything else that I was doing. I didn't ever feel like stopping it. I didn't do it because I had to, I did it because I wanted to. Somewhere at the back of my mind, I knew that even though this one prayer wasn't answered, God was still using me in many different areas to bless others.

February 2019 – It's not about you, it's about who God is

At the beginning of 2019, one of my New Year's resolutions was to stop moping about. I disliked feeling sorry for myself. I disliked it every time I spiralled down into a rabbit hole whenever I heard news of someone else's pregnancy. Desperate for a change, I told God I was going to let it go and let Him do whatever He wanted to.

Come to think of it, it really isn't about me. It's not what I have achieved. It's not that I have not received what God has promised me. It's not about what I have and don't have. It's not about me. It's never about me. It is about God. The Bible says many things about God, and I simply cannot list everything without quoting more than half the Bible. But I want to point out a couple of things.

God is love. If He is love, why would He promise me something and not give it to me? Does someone you love want you to suffer? Would someone you love like to see you sad all the time? More than that, if God has promised, isn't He capable of fulfilling His promises? He is able to, and He wants to. No matter what His promises are and what my requests are, He is able to. And that's all that should matter. That God is able to.

There was a shift in my mindset from then. It was no longer about me that mattered, but it was about God. It was about who God is, and who He is in my life. He is my Father who loves me, cares for me and is able to. I must say, since then my heart became lighter. Much lighter.

I had set up a few reminders around me to guide me should I fall back to my old ways, as I'm infamously known for my impatience. I changed my phone screen to reflect that, so that I would be reminded each time I looked at my phone.

The first time I heard "Way Maker" sung by Sinach, I was moved beyond my words can express. I wrote the lyrics on my mirror. I looked at them each time I walked in and out of that room, which was multiple times a day.

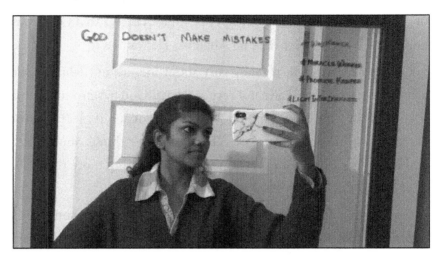

A blury picture of the lyrics of "Way Maker" on my mirror.

July 2019 – It's going to be OK

With the busyness of the new year at work, it was successful for a short period of time. I promptly forgot about my own resolution two months into the year. I slowly reverted to my old ways of moping about and sulking month after month. Let's just say I went back to being miserable on the inside whenever I was in my closet. On the outside, I looked perfect and confident. On the inside I was a complete wreck.

Somewhere around July 2019, I was reminded of a conversation I had with my senior pastor from church, Pastor Steve McEwen, and his wife, Anoushca, exactly a year ago to the date. They had invited us to their place for lunch one day to catch up. The agenda was obviously to talk about where we stood regarding expanding our family and to pray for us, but I carefully avoided that until the end of the day. When the topic did come up, most of my thoughts came pouring out. Only most. I very cautiously omitted to share with them about the promise and only mentioned about our plight with the healthcare system, and how we had not come to any conclusion at all.

After a few words of encouragement and prayers, Anoushca offered to be available for me as much as I needed. As much as I was grateful for her offer, I declined it. I refused to be vulnerable to someone else. I told her very openly that I would not be taking up the offer at all, but I truly appreciated her thoughts and prayers. When we were about to leave, Anoushca very specifically mentioned to me multiple times that it was going to be OK.

When we got back home that night, I psychoanalysed the afternoon, and I was fixated on "It's going to be OK". As much as I wanted to believe it, I couldn't. How could someone else know it's going to be OK?

My postgraduate degree in Psychology has rewired my brain to never use the phrase "it's going to be OK". According to Psychology, we never know if someone who is suffering will ever be OK. We are in no position to either confirm or deny that to the affected individuals, even if we have experienced the same issue. Everyone goes through different circumstances and has different reactions. Psychology believes that it gives false hope since we cannot predict the future, therefore saying "It's going to be OK" is not acceptable and rather counterproductive. We can only empathise but not confirm or deny any potential recovery. Ever since learning about this, I've never used those words to anyone else when I've been in a position of counselling. The only kind of reassuring I could ever give was that we would find some ways to manage their circumstances.

Managing is a far cry from everything being OK. Maybe it was because of this mindset that I wasn't able to accept and practise Anoushca's words straightaway. It was always running in my mind though, it just had not found a place to inhabit in my brain, because my brain was only functioning on the limited capacity that I had allowed it to.

A year on, I finally started finding hope in those words.

It's going to be OK. I can carry on with my life even if it hasn't panned out the way I think it should have been.

It's going to be OK. I can live my life without putting a stop to everything I wanted to do.

It's going to be OK. I don't have to put my life on hold.

It's going to be OK. I can travel for work.

It's going to be OK. I can go on holidays.

It's going to be OK. I can smile and be happy.

It's going to be OK. I know who holds my future.

It's going to be OK, especially when I do not have answers.

Why the sudden change of heart you ask? Psychology only says that man cannot predict the future. It never said anything about God. Unlike Psychology, I believed in God, a God who wants nothing but the best for me. A mere person cannot predict one's future, but God can. When you realise that, everything changes.

Watching the calendar

Over the years, I was diligently watching the calendar and counting the dates. I used several apps to track these things. I would be careful not to work out or over stress myself with work during certain times of the month. I turned down multiple work opportunities to travel and timed my holidays.

Months turned to years. By end of 2019, I gave up. I'd had enough with it. I'd had enough of thinking about nothing but this 24/7. I got fed up putting my life on hold, although I considered pregnancy as my life back then. It's funny how life changed for me from not thinking about children at all to being consumed by nothing but thoughts about having a baby.

Why was I so obsessed with it?

I felt like the promise did nothing for me other than add pressure. Promise = Pressure. It wasn't what I anticipated, nor was I a happy bunny.

I was fixated on it ever since I had heard that promise from God in August 2015. If God had promised something, it would be nothing but the best and I wanted that. I wanted the promise from God. Maybe not even so much about wanting a baby or being a mother. It was the gift from God that I was after.

Pressure from those around me was immensely infuriating. Sometimes I felt like I just wanted to have a baby so people would stop asking. It's not a good enough reason to want to have a child, but I cannot even describe enough how bad the pressure was for me. To the extent that I avoided family gatherings and social events like the plague. Funny how the metaphor of plagues worked out for me in both doubt and avoidance.

Old diary entries

I started logging my thoughts in relation to the promise in bits and pieces on my phone and laptop from time to time, right from 2016 until 2020. But I never thought these entries would see the light of day, therefore never organised them like I would normally do. However, at some point in my frustration, I had deleted some of the entries because I no longer wanted to recollect anything.

When I was prompted time and time again to write this book, I scouted out and found some still saved in places that I hadn't remembered I noted down.

Behold, ladies and gentlemen, you are about to enter my deepest and darkest place, where no one has ever set foot before . . .

29/03/2019

Will I make a good mother?

I find babies really cute and cuddly. But I also find changing nappies and caring for a sick baby impossible.

Why do I want to have a baby then?

How do I even have the guts to wish for this?

There's some sort of a connection. Some unexplainable bond. There's a desire. More than a desire, there's a yearning. It's so deep that it hurts a lot.

25/05/2019

Some friends said we will be very good at growing life. I can barely even keep a plant alive for more than a week. Surely they had no idea what they meant.

21/06/2019

On the flight on our way back to Glasgow to visit family and the arrival of a new baby, and I broke down uncontrollably. I didn't want to face anyone.

Why do I want to become a mother? I still haven't got an answer for it.

28/07/2019

We are at the church family camp. By now, three people have said that we'll make good parents.

01/09/2019

It was my turn on the rota to help in kids' church today. I've always got my reservations with other people's children, so I'm extra careful on how I talk to them. It usually takes me slightly longer to warm up to them.

Today, though, I found myself drawing to them quickly and warming up with them quickly. Everyone was excitedly talking about going back to school next week. Some of the kids were looking forward to it, some weren't. Some of the mothers in the room were talking about their kids' school uniform colours, etc.

I was extremely saddened that I don't have my own child yet.

22/09/2019

God is in the details. He doesn't make mistakes.

19/01/2020

I've been thinking for several months now if it's even worth logging anything. What's the point? I know in my spirit that I had to log it, but my mind doesn't agree. Who's going to read it? Where is all this going to go?

I recalled something that someone once told me that God allows you to go through something so you can counsel those who have the same experience now. She shared her experience of going through breast cancer so she could counsel her friend who was in the same situation.

Is this what God is trying to tell me?

28/08/2020

Seven months since I last made a conscious effort to log my thoughts. Maybe I didn't want to recall them anymore? Perhaps I no longer want to remember, or relive the experience? Did I lose hope? Did I lose faith in the promise that God had given me? Sometimes the answer to that is a resounding yes, other times it's a no. I don't know what else life means without faith in God.

I wouldn't blame you if you had even the slightest bit of judgement towards me while reading the above. At this point, I no longer care what anyone thought about me or my secrets. When I read my own thoughts, I didn't even know what to make out of it myself. I was in a complete mess most of the time.

I couldn't help but notice how I penned my thoughts for years whenever I felt defeated. But the day I found out I was pregnant, I was so completely at a loss for words that I did not write anything, nor did I write much after that.

In some of the entries, I was so cynical that it sounded like I wanted to jot down my thoughts only so I had evidence to prove to God when I had a go at Him. Having a row with God isn't foreign behaviour to me anyway. But in real life, I'm not a pessimist.

56

Why not IVF?

I strongly believe that every child is God breathed. It is God who gives life, regardless of whether it was a natural conception or with a little help from science. It is God who gives wisdom to scientists to figure out such methods in the first place.

Having said that, I had nothing against IVF, except for the fact that the process itself was so daunting to me that I had no guts whatsoever to pursue it. I kept putting it off as much as I could. Knowing me, if it were to be something that I so badly wanted, I wouldn't think twice about the process. But this wasn't the same. Laxman was sitting on the fence about it partially because of me because I wasn't a hundred per cent willingly into it. Ultimately it would be me who had to suffer the physical consequences of the whole process of IVF and not him. He was also hesitant mostly because he didn't have the peace. He didn't want me to pull a Sarah[6] to build a family in my own way when he knew that God Himself would intervene. We were praying for God's perfect will to happen and didn't want to take matters into our own hands and disrupt what God was doing.

When we were told that our last and final option was IVF, I was nervous about the process. When we were told that we wouldn't receive any funding and we would need to fork out all the money, I was even more doubtful. To the extent that we kept putting it off multiple times. Also, the fact that IVF's success rate was less than 50 per cent was even more daunting. So, it was not even guaranteed that we would definitely conceive if we were to do IVF. There's so many scientific explanations and statistics that say IVF success rates increase with multiple tries. There was no way we would be able to go through repeat cycles with all the emotional, physical and financial toll that comes along with it.

Doubts started creeping in

By now, it's no secret that doubt took the better of me uncountable times during those five years that I was waiting. If I were to be given a penny for every time I questioned God about it, I would be rich by now.

How many times can I tell my mother off that I don't want to talk about it? How many times can I avoid my mother-in-law every time she wants to make herbal food to help with fertility?

I wanted to tell people to stop. But I couldn't. I wanted to yell at the top of my voice every time I heard it, but I couldn't. Well, I have a few times until some got the message and stopped, while others didn't get the memo and insisted on repeating it. Doesn't anyone understand that asking me the question doesn't miraculously make me pregnant?

Every time someone questioned me, I was humiliated.

Why haven't you had any children yet?

The clock is ticking.

Are you trying?

Did you see the doctor?

You've been married for so many years and still don't have any children. My daughter got married last year and has a son now.

Are you taking any medication?

Someone I know took folic acid, and they got pregnant immediately.

Are you doing any treatments?

You need to put on more weight to carry a baby.

When are you going to tell us the good news?

I wished the earth would swallow me, or better still them, so I wouldn't have to face them. Laxman usually tried to remind me that it came from a place of concern. Yeah, some did, some didn't, but none of these questions are OK, even if it comes from a place of concern and love. I was humiliated every time I had to say I wasn't pregnant, or that I did not know when I would be because it was not in my control. I wasn't going to tell anyone that I'd done hundreds of blood tests and investigations, but doctors couldn't find anything wrong.

These things triggered me to doubt the promise that I was holding on to.

Did I actually hear God correctly?

Maybe it was just in my mind.

It's a very common verse that everyone uses. Surely God didn't mean it for me.

As the months and years passed, the plague of doubt grew beyond my control. I couldn't find answers anywhere. I obviously hadn't shared this promise with anyone else, so I couldn't even go to anyone else. Anyhow, with something so important like this about my life and future, God would speak to me directly first and not to or through others.

To make matters worse, I was singing songs in church like "I will put my trust in you, and I will not be shaken". Really? I wanted to mean it, but I couldn't. I sang like I meant it, but I knew deep down I was still fighting with God. Such words are so much more easily sung than practised in real life.

Faith can be foggy sometimes because you cannot see the future. But in all seriousness, I mean every word of it. It felt like too much time had passed for the promise to be true, especially with the silence from God throughout those years.

If you were looking for some sort of solace from my coping mechanisms, I'm sorry to say that I didn't have very healthy ones back then. My coping strategies changed from time to time. It started off with questioning, avoiding, fighting, and overeating. Then took a sharp turn towards healthy eating along with exercising very regularly. I threw myself into it. I had goals to achieve, which I did and became the fittest and healthiest I had ever been, and yet none of it satisfied me. Ultimately, I surrendered to God which, in hindsight, I should have done right from day one. Deep down I knew I couldn't change anything.

From my experience, I can advise you of something that I didn't do myself, but so badly wished I did. I was too full of myself and wanted to be more hands-on in everything. So, I had to stick my impatient self into it and ruin my own peace of mind. I would highly recommend a large serving of peace for breakfast, lunch, and dinner, seasoned generously with patience, and topped off with a sprinkle of joy. For snacks, please have some openness to listening to God. And you can wash it all down with some courage in the things you cannot see but confidence in the one who is in complete control.

The Push

My fear about pregnancy and labour

A couple of months into my pregnancy, I was recommended a book, *Supernatural Childbirth* by Jackie Mize. Reading that book gave me a revelation I wouldn't have thought of otherwise. *I could actually pray for painless delivery?*

In her book, Jackie spoke about the difference between natural birth and supernatural birth. Jackie says, "In natural childbirth classes there are exercises. The woman is taught to centre in on a focal point, to pant and breathe as directed and the husband is taught to coach her through it. When I refer to supernatural childbirth, I'm talking strictly about being able to conceive and to have babies with a pregnancy free from nausea, morning sickness, pain, moodiness, depression and without fear of any kind; then going through the entire labour without pain, and through the delivery without stiches and anaesthetic. I'm talking about using the Word of God to overcome, change and make things better."[7]

My experience was nothing supernatural as per the definition above, but it made a whole world of a difference in the way I prayed and viewed my pregnancy and labour.

My biggest fear around pregnancy was always the labour and changing nappies. They are in no way equal, but to me, they triggered a lot of anxiety. As a result, I was very careful not to look at any childbirth videos on YouTube or read too much into it. I only learnt the science and basics of it and nothing more than that. When it was time to prepare my birth plan, out of the multiple pain relief options, I made up my mind that I was going to opt for gas and air (Entonox) as a pain relief tool. It is a mixture of oxygen and nitrous oxide gas that doesn't remove the pain completely but helps reduce it, making it more manageable. You can breathe in the air through a mask or mouthpiece that is handheld, controlled by yourself. Other than that, I was more than willing to have a caesarean if needed. In fact, I would have opted for a C-section from the very beginning had I been offered a choice! I was happy for any medical intervention if needed during the process.

The day I went into labour

Let me tell you my labour story so you understand where I'm coming from. It's a funny one and I promise I'll spare you the gory details. I love telling this story, or rather recalling it, because it was truly a light-hearted moment both during the labour and even afterwards. Some may say it was the Entonox gas, but I know it was the Holy Spirit.

I woke up on 13th April 2021 at about 4am to go to the loo. That was my body's natural alarm throughout my pregnancy. When I got back to bed, I couldn't sleep. It was such a common recurrence throughout my pregnancy that I got accustomed to it, so I just laid in bed hoping I would eventually be able to go back to sleep. But something felt very different that morning.

The night before, Levi was unusually active in my tummy. Ever since week twenty of my pregnancy, his usual play time was about 9-10pm when I got into bed and started relaxing. That was his cue for playtime. He loved kicking about and always played with Laxman. Every time Laxman nudged into my belly in different positions, Levi would turn around to kick his hand back. The two of them would be having a game of football for a good thirty minutes sometimes.

On the twelfth night, though, his kicks were far stronger and more frequent than ever before. We even thought he might kick his way out through my belly at the rate he was going. Which was what led me to feel different the next morning.

It was as if I was unconsciously anticipating something. Within twenty minutes I had a pain and, in that instant, I knew it was a contraction. This was a constant thought in my mind towards the end of my pregnancy. How does a contraction really feel? If it is like regular cramps, what if I miss it? What if it isn't strong enough? No matter how much someone else explains it to you, there is no way you can comprehend it until you experience it yourself. Well, my first contraction wasn't very strong, but I knew it was a contraction for sure. I reached out for my phone and clicked into the contraction tracker app and noted the first one. Nothing happened for the next couple of minutes, but I was even more alert now if I wasn't awake enough before.

Ten minutes later, my waters broke! It was like a small gush of water and I knew for sure it was my waters and not that I had peed myself. This was another thing I was always concerned about. I sat up in bed and waited, not knowing what I was waiting for, but I waited for another ten or fifteen minutes before waking Laxman. I had mild and irregular contractions within that time, and my waters were leaking slowly but surely. When I told Laxman my waters had broken and I felt some contractions, he bounced out of bed, got dressed and was ready to leave right that minute!

When in labour, we were told that the procedure would be to monitor contractions and call the hospital if the waters broke. We gave it about half an hour and called the delivery suite at about 5am, while still in bed. The midwife took a few details from me and told me to monitor my contractions and call them back if the frequency or intensity increased.

After the call, we both sat in bed and tried to remain calm. I was somewhat OK, trying to figure out what was next. Laxman, however, was on extra alert mode. A few minutes later, I got up from bed for the first time since 4am to take a shower and get ready for the day. It no longer felt like I was going to be able to go back to sleep that morning. The minute I set foot in the shower, my waters broke fully. There was a big gush of water that was flowing through non-stop.

I've always wondered if this experience would really be like how it is in the movies, and what I would do if I were to be out and about when my waters broke. Thank God it was while I was in my shower and not while I was outdoors. And thank God it wasn't even so bad while I was still in bed. Otherwise, I would have been thinking about changing my bedsheets instead of getting to the hospital! I stood in the shower and called out to Laxman. It just wouldn't stop but contractions were still the same, mild and irregular. I had to call the midwife immediately from in the shower. The midwife told me to come into the hospital because they would need to start monitoring now the waters had fully broken.

I still didn't rush though; I took my time to have my shower while Laxman woke my mother up and told her that my waters had broken and that we were going to go to the hospital. Once I got out of the shower, my mother and Laxman were nervously waiting for me, while I wanted to get ready. As in, I wanted to get dressed properly and put on some make-up to look presentable. My idea of make-up includes some eye liner and blusher. Both my mother and Laxman were looking at me as if I had lost the plot. They insisted that I needed to get to the hospital as soon as possible instead of thinking about dressing up. It was 6am, and by the sound of the midwife on the phone, and the fact that my waters had broken fully and felt like they were fully drained, I thought the baby was going to come anytime soon. I wanted to look presentable for pictures once baby arrived. How naïve I was! This is nothing short of a classic first-time mother experience.

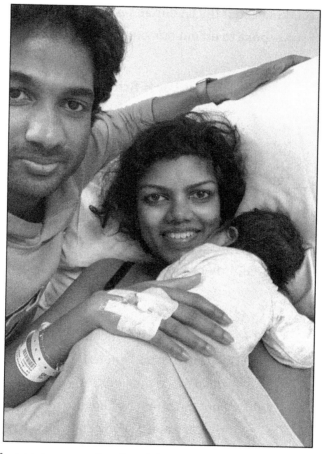

Our first picture as a family of three at 6pm. Not the look I was aiming for when I tried to put on some make-up at 6am to look presentable.

Hospital assessment centre

The drive from our home to the hospital was only ten minutes during off-peak hours. We had already done a trial run and we knew exactly how long it would take us to get there, and even had a song ready for the ten-minute journey. Tauren Wells' "Famous For" (Wells, 2020) was playing on repeat mode while we drove, both in silence. I was nervous thinking about the labour and so was Laxman. Every word from that song spoke to us and our situation.

Famous For (I Believe)[8]

There is no fear 'cause I believe
There is no doubt 'cause I have seen
Your faithfulness, my fortress, over and over

I have a hope found in Your name
I have a strength found in Your grace
Your faithfulness, my fortress, over and over

Make way through the waters
Walk me through the fire
Do what You are famous for,
what You are famous for
Shut the mouths of lions
Bring dry bones to life and
Do what You are famous for,
what You are famous for
I believe in You
God, I believe in You

Release Your love inside of me
Unleash Your power for all to see Spirit, come, and fall on us
Over and over, oh Lord

God of exceedingly, God of abundantly
More than we ask or think
Lord, You will never fail
Your name is powerful, Your word's unstoppable
All things are possible in You

There is no fear 'cause I believe
There is no doubt 'cause I have seen
Your faithfulness, my fortress, over and over

We reached the hospital at about 6.15am. I was told that I needed to go to the assessment unit through a different entrance instead of the actual delivery ward, and that I would have to go alone, while Laxman waited in the car. By now my contractions had increased, both in intensity and frequency.

Laxman walked with me to the entrance, and I stopped to take some pictures along the way because I wanted to remember everything on that day. *This is it! We are finally going to meet our baby.* I didn't want to forget anything. I wanted Laxman to take a picture of me before going in, but he refused to. He just wanted me to go in and get checked ASAP. Since he refused to take a picture of me, I took pictures of the entrance

The walk all the way from the entrance to the actual assessment unit was a very long, slow walk. I had to stop every couple of minutes to ride out the contractions. And to make matters worse, my waters were still leaking. How much amniotic fluid does the body carry? I waited for almost an hour for someone to attend to me. Apparently, it wasn't as urgent as I thought it might be.

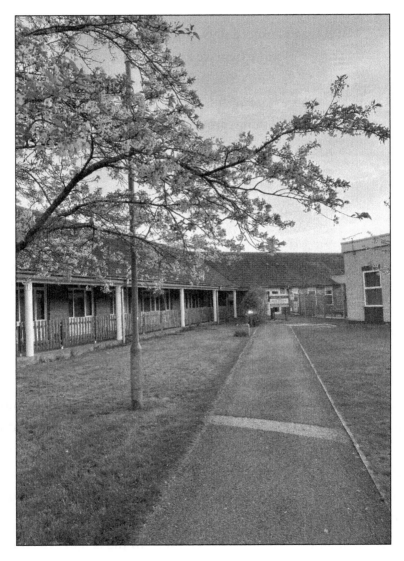

Picture of the entrance to remind Laxman that he refused to take a picture of me waddling in to the maternity unit to have our baby.

One midwife strapped me up to monitor baby's heartbeat, came back a couple of minutes later and said she would need to speak to a consultant as it looked like baby's heartbeat was slower than normal. She reappeared again a few minutes later and strapped me up to another machine and measured baby's heartbeat again. It still showed baby's heartbeat was slower than normal. But she told me not to worry and continued with their other procedures. Not easily done as told.

Contractions were surely increasing by then. When the midwife checked to see how much I was dilated, she looked rather shocked and went to get a doctor for a second opinion. Checking dilation is not a very pleasant experience. Imagine how much more unpleasant it is if there are two people checking it back-to-back! Turns out, I was already 7cm dilated and they had not expected that at all since I was still calm and didn't show any signs of being in pain or of having severe contractions.

Seemingly, someone who's 7cm dilated would probably be screaming in pain because contractions would already be very intense. To be honest, my contractions were more severe than at 5am, but they weren't as intense as they made it sound they should have been.

Trust me when I say they were not the only ones surprised. I have zero threshold to pain and didn't think I would survive with a smile when I was 7cm dilated. They were going to take me to the delivery suite ASAP and needed Laxman to get his lateral flow test done immediately so that he could come inside the delivery suite when I was taken in. I phoned Laxman and told him to do the lateral flow test ASAP otherwise he wouldn't be allowed in. By the sound of things from the doctor and midwife, it sounded like the baby would arrive in an hour or two. So I kind of rushed him, and Laxman was also in a shock that I was already 7cm dilated.

I thought they were going to wheel me to the delivery suite, but I had to walk there. It was another very long and painful walk. I had several contractions in that journey, therefore slowing me down.

Delivery suite

I don't know where the time had gone, but when I reached the delivery suite it was already 10.30am. Laxman was waiting for me just outside the room. We were taken to a room with an en-suite bathroom. But it wasn't one of those rooms with bathtub delivery and hypnobirthing, etc. They offered to change me to another room, but I didn't want any of those. Just give me a plain, simple, clinical room. I wanted to make sure we had all the support if there were to be any kind of emergency. I wasn't up for water birthing.

The midwife showed me around the room and let Laxman prop up my suitcase and settle in. She asked if I wanted an epidural or any other pain relief. I told her I was going to opt for gas and air, only if and when I needed it.

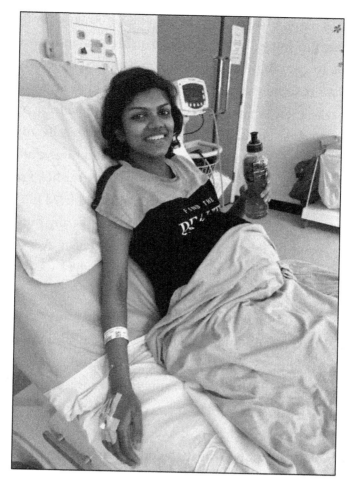

I was trying to get myself comfortable on the bed, but I felt uncomfortable regardless. The midwife suggested that it would help if I were to walk for a bit, so I was walking around the room. The pain started increasing gradually. For the first part, I was managing with the breathing techniques that I had learnt from my antenatal class and declined the offer of pain relief from the midwife. But that didn't last very long. She thought I was being so brave that I didn't need any pain relief. But I couldn't take it anymore by 12 noon.

After 12 noon, I had to take the gas and air because my breathing techniques no longer sufficed. When using gas and air, it is not advisable to constantly be on it. The midwife explained that using gas and air is somewhat equivalent to getting high on alcohol. You need to take a few breaths of gas and then get some fresh air, hence why it's called gas and air. I did just that for an hour. By 1pm, I was completely out. The pain escalated so quickly and I was clutching on to the tube of gas as if I was clutching on to my dear life. From then onwards, I closed my eyes shut to concentrate and tried not to focus on the pain. I could no longer open my eyes and see anything around me or respond to anyone properly, but I could hear everyone very clearly and I was fully alert. The midwife thought I was becoming semi unconscious, but I wasn't.

At 1.30pm, the midwife checked again and said I was still only 7cm dilated. Which means I hadn't dilated any more at all since morning. I was pretty disappointed to hear that! They suggested hormone drips to encourage further dilation, but the doctor wasn't available to do it immediately, so we had to keep going on our own. Laxman and I were actually pleased that the doctor wasn't available then, because I didn't want to be induced at all. It adds on to more unpleasantness. At 3.30pm the midwife checked again before going to find a doctor and announced that I was already 10cm dilated. It was finally time to push!

The labour

I was so pleased to hear that, and yet I thought I was already pushing earlier. During the contractions, I had the urge to push so I did. But deceptively that was only the contractions. I needed to start pushing for real now. I pushed and pushed with all my might, or so I thought.

But I couldn't feel any progress or movement from inside. In the half-drowsy state that I was in and while biting onto the gas tube, I tried to communicate by saying a few words, forming incoherent sentences, and everyone in the room had to make sense of what I was saying.

I told them I couldn't feel anything move and suggested they do a caesarean. I was worried about the baby because it had been so long and I heard someone say his heartbeat was decreasing slowly but it was still safe for him. The midwife laughed at my suggestion because the baby was too far down and that was the only way he could come out now. I continued pushing and pushing but there was no sign of the baby yet.

The normal procedure if the baby was struggling to pass through the birth canal due to his head being bigger than the space available, would be to do an incision called an episiotomy, followed by ventouse suction cups (works like a vacuum), followed by forceps. These are the only steps I have been made aware of, and these were all used on me. Where possible, it's best to avoid these as they could cause extra damage. I was terrified of having too much damage but that's exactly what happened.

I knew it even before the midwife said out loud that the baby's head was too big for me. They asked if I was OK with an episiotomy to help and minimise any tears. I agreed, not like I had any other choice then. I just wanted to do everything we could to get him out. The episiotomy didn't help enough. I had suggested the vacuum well before they even suggested an episiotomy to me. So, when the next question came about using the ventouse, I agreed immediately. They needed a doctor to do it and had paged for both a doctor and a consultant. The doctor arrived first around 4.30pm. When they were ready, the doctor gave me several instructions on what to do. Followed through, but it didn't work. When the doctor had the ventouse in position attached to baby's head that was crowning, all I heard was a pop and the whole room went quiet. That was the sound of the vacuum detaching from the baby's head. We started off at 10.30am with two midwives and Laxman and I. By 4.30pm, we ended up with several extras who had come in to support. There was pin-drop silence in a room that had been as noisy as a market just a few seconds before. Laxman said his heart stopped when that happened. I still had my eyes shut tight, so I couldn't see anything but I heard every single thing, and felt every emotion in the room. Nervous, tension, stress, worry, concerns. It all ultimately means only one thing – the baby is still inside, and his heartbeat was dropping slowly. Later I was also told that I was bleeding out due to the episiotomy. They needed to use the next tool to aid the labour. The consultant stepped in and asked if I was OK with them using forceps.

Yes, yes, yes, do anything you need to get the baby out, I'm not risking anything else.

The moment of birth

From the moment the consultant stepped in at about 5pm, it felt as if everything was on time-lapse mode. The consultant was very assertive and did not waste any time. From the minute she stepped in, she meant business. I heard clear and precise instructions about the tool and what would happen next.

Upon the consultant's instructions, the midwives had to force my fingers open to get the gas tube away from me and forced me to open my eyes and stay focused on pushing. She gave me instructions on when to push and when not to push so that she could insert the forceps and position them around the baby's head and get into position so we would work together. There was once when she told me not to push, I snapped back at her saying I couldn't help it, I needed to push now!

A few twists and turns of the forceps and she was ready for me to push while she was pulling. When she was pulling the baby out, they forced me to open my eyes, because I still had them shut tight. She asked me to look, and I remember opening my eyes and telling her I couldn't see anything, because I really couldn't see anything beyond my bump, and I didn't even feel any wriggling in my belly. She then pulled the baby out and lifted him out, and I finally saw him. She plopped him on my tummy immediately. He was big and heavy and adorable, despite being covered in all the gunge.

The whole room was no longer relevant to me. I had completely forgotten about my surrounding. I couldn't hear anyone else talking, I didn't see the commotion in the room.

I only had eyes for Levi. Born at 5.09pm on 13th April, weighing all of 3.4kg, with a head full of hair, big brown eyes, button nose, small ears, wiggly and ever so interested in his new surroundings that he was calmly staring at everyone and everything.

This is the baby I had not even dreamt of but was so desperate for. The pain of labour had no effect on me at that moment. I was still bleeding out, but it bothered me the least bit.

I now have a child. I have a son. Can you believe it? I couldn't!

Stitching up

A few minutes later, the midwife wanted to take him away to get him cleaned and dressed up. I didn't know it was a midwife who was trying to pick him up; I thought he was sliding away from my tummy since he was so heavy. I tightened my grip around him, and it became a bit of a tug-of-war between me and her. She thought I was still high and didn't know what I was doing, but I was fully aware that I was holding on to the baby thinking he was sliding away. She then explained to me that they were going to clean him up and dress him up. She took him away to the corner of the room where they had an area set up for new-born babies.

Laxman went with them to watch what they were doing.

At this point, the consultant had to leave, so the doctor stepped in. Since I'd had an episiotomy and a second-degree tear, I had to have a lot of stitches. The doctor offered two options. The first was to move me to another room and give me an epidural through my spine so that I didn't feel anything during the procedure. This would take longer given the logistics, etc. The second option was to do the stitches there and then in the same room. I didn't want an epidural right from the beginning, so it would have defeated the purpose of declining it for labour and having it done now, so I naturally picked option two, which was to have it done in the same room, provided I could have the gas and air to help with pain relief.

I figured they were hoping for me to choose option two because they let out a sigh of relief and laughed when I asked if I could keep the gas and air. It was a better option according to them as it wouldn't be safe to delay it.

So much for gas and air to the rescue. I was biting and screaming through the tube for the entirety of the procedure of stitching.

The overall experience

Throughout the labour, I was very surprised with myself by how calm and collected I was right from the beginning till the end. Well, for most of it. Even when I was high on gas and air, I was still aware of everything and, despite the intensity, I could joke with the midwives.

A few things that could go wrong did go wrong. A lot of things that I didn't want to happen had happened – I had to wait on my own in the assessment centre, waiting nervously for the midwife to check with a consultant whether the baby's heartbeat monitor was a true reflection of the baby's heartbeat or not. Having to go through two membrane sweeps one after another to confirm I was definitely 7cm dilated. During labour, my contractions progressed in a couple of hours, but the dilation hadn't. I didn't want to be induced but the midwives had already requested for me to be induced and were waiting for the doctor to come. I ended up with an episiotomy when that was one of the things I didn't want to happen, along with a tear. During active labour, not only did the ventouse not work, it popped out, leaving my baby stuck inside. As a final resort, the consultant had to step in and use forceps. I wasn't against this, but I would have preferred not to use these tools. The use of such tools can cause higher chances of infection both for mother and baby.

On the surface, the entire labour seemed chaotic and nerve wrecking, but all I remember from it was having a laugh and even providing some entertainment for the medical staff in the room while I was in labour. I would like to think that it wasn't all credit to the gas and air.

There was certainly a fair share of experiences shared with me that labour is pretty traumatic. It left me wondering why anyone would be willing to have consecutive children if they found it so traumatising the first time round. Having had things done in a rush and having the added pressure that the baby's heartbeat was dropping, and that I was bleeding out, I wasn't traumatised.

It feels strange to put it down in writing when that was exactly one of my biggest concerns from the very beginning. In fact, Laxman was probably the one who was traumatised. During my labour, I developed some muscle cramps in my calf muscles and feet. These muscle cramps are quite a normal occurrence for me and Laxman knows what to do to help relieve them because he's done it hundreds of times before at home. None of the midwives understood my cramps and couldn't help me. I had a big belly and was in labour, so I couldn't do anything myself. Laxman was the only other person who knew what to do and stepped in. He was sat by my shoulder in the beginning, as every birth partner is expected to, feeding me isotonic drink from my water bottle. But then he moved to my feet to help me out with the cramps. Birth partners are usually not allowed at the feet during labour, but none of us could help the situation. He obviously had a front row seat to all the action that was going on. While I experienced birth physically, he had an eyeful of it. It took him a good couple of weeks to forget the whole picture (. . . or maybe not).

I really hope you don't feel like I am boasting when I say I didn't feel any pain. And it definitely feels weird to share it, but I feel obliged to. This is such a surreal experience for me that I am not sure how it happened. Sure, it took me six weeks to recover from all the stitches and the actual labour. Yes, I was screaming and yelling between 1pm-6pm. I did apologise to everyone in the room in advance and after. As soon as the stiches were done, I no longer felt any pain. And the biggest surprise I had was that I didn't cry throughout the entire labour. I only shed emotional tears when I saw Laxman carrying Levi after he was cleaned and dressed up. I didn't even realise this until Laxman pointed it out to me later that night.

Deep down in my heart, I thought I would give up halfway during labour and something was going to go wrong. I had no idea I would be able to cope with it. Not crying during labour through everything is a miracle even for me. I have zero threshold to pain. If you so much as flick me, I will flinch in pain.

Someone told me that women usually step-up during labour as the time calls for it. I know for a fact that it wasn't me. It isn't normal according to my standards to not cry while going through so much pain. It isn't in my nature to be calm from the beginning and not lose my cool given the circumstances I was in. I will say it again, it wasn't me. It wasn't the hormones. It wasn't the gas and air.

It was God.

If it wasn't for His intervention, I would have completely lost it when the baby wasn't budging despite trying to push my insides out. The minute I heard the ventouse pop out empty, and the baby's heartbeat was dropping, I would have panicked and had a meltdown.

Simply put, if it wasn't for God, I wouldn't be writing this chapter and you wouldn't be reading it.

The Pride

When I came back home from the hospital a day later, I received what felt like a warrior's welcome. My family had decorated the house to welcome Levi and me. There was healthy homemade herbal soup waiting for me because I'd hardly eaten anything for two days. My mother welcomed me saying, "Well done." (I don't remember the last time she said those words to me directly.) My mother-in-law said I was very resilient. My in-laws and nieces were so excited and happy. Those gestures truly made me feel like a warrior, like I had achieved something no one else had and that I deserved all the praises. It felt like I deserved it, all of it!

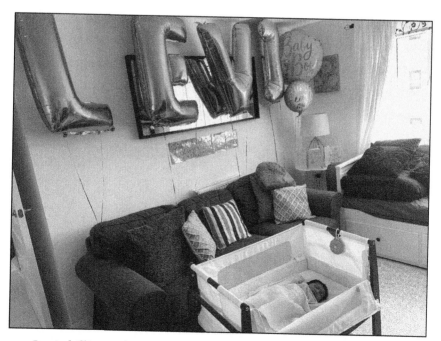

Levi chilling at home amongst his Welcome Home decorations.

But from the very bottom of my heart, I knew I didn't. It wasn't my own doing, and it most definitely wasn't pride on my part to deserve any of it.

I chose to name this chapter The Pride mainly because it had a nice ring to it and went well along with the rest of the chapters. But I am truly proud of something that I want to share. I'm not good at accepting compliments or making a statement that/when I am right. So, bear with me while I try to waffle through and explain it as best as I can.

There were many moments during the pregnancy where Laxman and I had our own doubts but never shared them with each other, in hope of not increasing any more anxiety for each other. It started right from the very first day of finding out we were pregnant at about four weeks. I went through all my skin care items, trying to make sure each was pregnancy safe and that none of the ingredients in them would pose any sort of risk to the pregnancy.

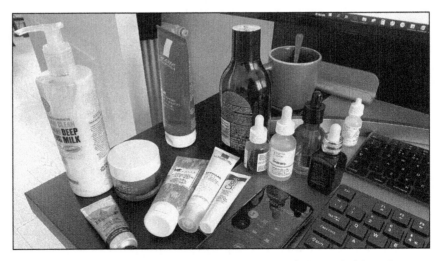

Checking skin care safety during pregnancy while on hold with GP.

At seven weeks, I had a case of bleeding. It was more like heavy spotting, but I didn't know the difference so I panicked, couldn't calm down and ended up at the emergency antenatal clinic for a scan, where the midwife reassured me that the pregnancy was safe and that there was nothing to worry about, although she couldn't explain the bleeding.

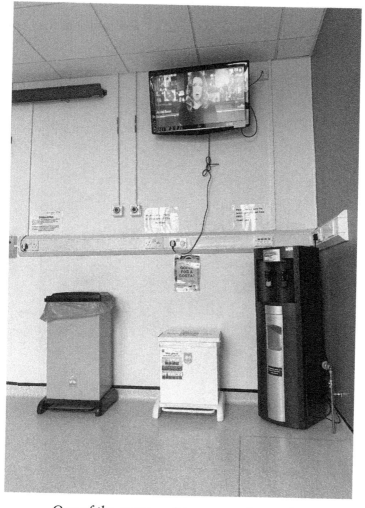

One of the many waiting rooms I've sat in.

At about thirty-two weeks pregnant, I went to A&E with a case of green morning sickness. What should have been the regular morning sickness that I'd endured since the beginning of pregnancy was different that day because it was bright green in colour, which I knew wasn't normal. But after having sat in the A&E for four hours on Valentine's Day morning, being transferred from one department to another, doing multiple blood tests and urine tests, (while Laxman was in the car park because of Covid), I was told that they couldn't explain anything and that everything looked normal.

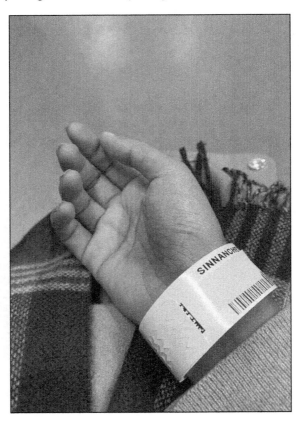

Spending Valentine's day and my Sunday morning in A&E waiting to be told there's nothing wrong

Since it took us so long to get pregnant, I was naturally over thinking everything and was over sensitive to any changes that my body went through. I would google every tiny symptom or read between the lines. I didn't want to miss anything in hope that I could nip it in the bud. Let's just say I was being paranoid. For someone who was so over controlling about the pregnancy, my decision to not do a screening test at twelve weeks was rather shocking even to myself.

Twelve-week scan

The NHS in England offers a dating scan and a screening test at around the twelfth week of pregnancy. The dating scan is to check how far along the pregnancy is, the estimated due date, to ensure baby is growing in the right place, and to check baby's development, while the screening test is to check for certain chromosomal disorders like Down's syndrome, Edwards' syndrome and Patau's syndrome. The initial screening test will show if the pregnancy is at high risk or low risk. If identified as high risk, the expectant couples will be offered more tests to find out for certain if the baby has those conditions and, if the situation calls for it, termination of the pregnancy.

Many people react differently to this. The screening test is optional but more often than not, people think it's a standard procedure so feel obliged to do it.

I for one had made up my mind that I didn't want to do the screening test at any cost. I was at the age where it was most likely going to turn out high risk, after which I would be invited to speak to a consultant to do more tests. If it did turn out as high risk with complications, I didn't want to spend the rest of my pregnancy worrying about what would happen next. Laxman and I knew that we wouldn't terminate the pregnancy regardless of what the results would be. While I had made my choice, I asked Laxman multiple times leading up to that day if he wanted to do the screening or if he was fine not doing it. Each time his answer was, "No, we don't have to do it." Nothing more than that, no explanations, no reasoning. So I never knew if he decided not to do it for my own peace of mind since I didn't want to do it, or if he himself didn't want to do it because he, too, wouldn't agree to a termination if offered.

When the day came, we were more excited to see the baby in the ultrasound scan and hadn't really given much thought about the screening. When the midwife asked to confirm what we were getting done that day, I confidently told her that we were only doing the dating scan and not the screening tests. During the scan, Laxman and I were in awe looking at the screen. A very wiggly baby was kicking around and even turned around to face the scanning device as if he was looking at us through the screen. The very sight of an active baby at twelve weeks put us at ease. The midwife said he was so active that she had hardly seen any other babies like that. My heart was so full of pride. Thinking back now, I feel she might have said that to many other pregnant women because it's just a harmlessly nice thing to say to expectant parents.

We had never come this far before. To be able to experience this was a whole new world of joy and peace. Nothing else mattered to us.

Twenty-week screening scan

The second scan during pregnancy is around twenty weeks. This is a screening scan which is optional too. This scan is a more detailed one to check the physical development of the baby. They check measurements for baby's head circumference, length and legs and feet, spinal cord, belly, kidneys, heart valves functioning the right way, and weight.

It is also during this scan that the NHS will offer a gender scan. Laxman and I were too impatient to wait until the twentieth week, so we did a private scan at sixteen weeks to find out the gender. I'm so glad we did, because on the morning of the twenty-week scan appointment, we were told at the reception desk that Laxman would not be allowed inside due to the new Covid restrictions. He ended up having to go back to wait in the car. Had we not done the private scan, he wouldn't have experienced seeing the baby again.

I chose to do the twenty-week scan because I was too fixated on the gender scan and didn't even realise the rest of the baby measurements taken were for screening purposes. I also obviously wanted to see the baby as much as I could. During the scan, the midwife confirmed the baby's gender, and proceeded to do the rest of the measurements.

I cannot lie, but I was extremely nervous during this appointment. I didn't want anything to be wrong, but since we had waited for so long, it was almost like we were waiting for something to go wrong, especially when we let our guard down. The midwife must have sensed my nervousness; she confirmed to me after each measurement that it was perfect.

At the end of the appointment, after what felt like the longest time ever, the midwife smiled at me and said everything was perfect. This little baby was perfect, just perfect. I walked out from the room lightheaded. This is exactly what I had been praying for: for this baby to be perfect in God's eyes and in man's eyes. She may not know it and she could have been describing most babies in the same way, but to me it made a whole world of a difference.

While I sat waiting for them to update my maternity book, I texted Laxman to say that everything was perfect. That's all I said. Laxman was overjoyed when he received that text. That's exactly what he was praying for too. His prayer was for the baby to be perfect. Later that day, he told me that it was one of the words he had used every morning while he was praying for the baby. We never told each other that we were praying for perfection, but we were praying for the same thing individually, unknown to each other.

Deciding on the name

From the very beginning of announcing our baby's gender, a lot of people started asking us if we had a name. That was a tough bullet to dodge. There was so much pressure about naming him. Once again, it boiled down to the fact that we were finally pregnant after such a long time, that everyone expected so much out of that pregnancy and for that baby. It felt like the name had to be perfect. Not just a good name, or a suitable name, it had to be a perfect name!

As if everyone asking and giving suggestions wasn't enough pressure, we also had to consider the fact that we needed a name that suited both our Asian family and the local culture that we live in too. From the day we did our gender scan at sixteen weeks, Laxman and I started thinking of names individually and would input them into a shared document we had in Notion. We would put the name along with its origin and meaning. Once we had several names, we would discuss their pros and cons together. Laxman wanted a name that started with the letter L because both our official names start with L.

I wasn't too fussed about the initial. I just wanted a name that suited him and meant the right thing for him.

We had a few names in our pot and we were toying around with some of them. We would even attempt to use that name when we were playing with the baby while he was kicking about in the womb. Sometimes he would respond to the names and that made us more excited. More than his response, we knew that the right name would definitely click with us right away. We both spent hours searching for names in the Bible and online. We did tons of research about names. We just wanted the perfect name, not just a popular one that had a nice ring to it. It had to suit him, and it had to live up to the family's expectations. If it didn't, I knew we wouldn't hear the end of it!

While I contributed several names to the pot, there was one name in particular that was really close to me, but I just wasn't too sure. I'd had the name in my mind for about five years – Levi. Yes, it was the same amount of time since I'd had the promise that we would have a son. A couple of months after the original promise, God told me that he would be called Levi. And the name has stayed on with me. I never spoke to Laxman about this.

I sneakily included the name Levi in the pot and we were discussing it. Laxman kind of grew fond of that name over all the other names. For one it started with L, and secondly, he had some sort of a connection with the name that he couldn't explain. He did a lot of his own research about the name.

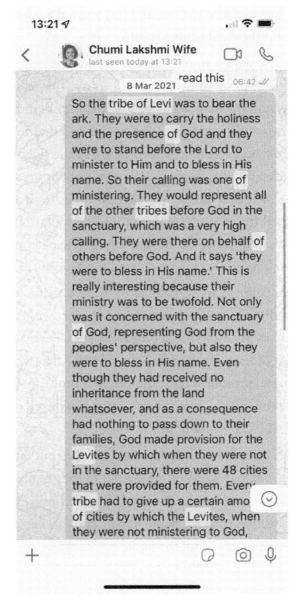

Laxman's text to me with his research about what Levi meant

In March 2021, Laxman celebrated me for Mother's Day even though I hadn't given birth yet. He bought me a Mother's Day card and said on it that he and Levi were very blessed to have me.

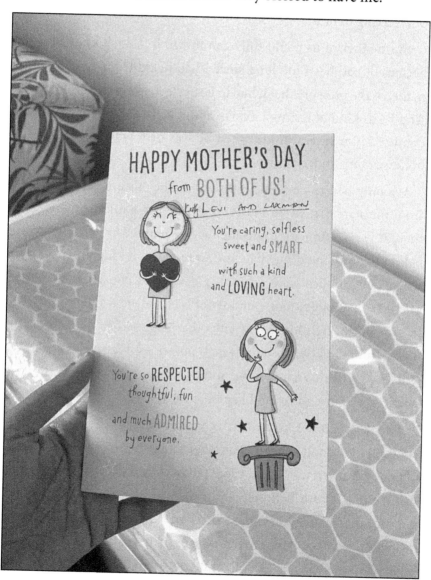

My very first mother's day card

That was a done deal for me. It was in writing now, so it had to be real. Amongst all the other names that we tried to use while I was still pregnant, Levi was the one we used the most while playing with him or referring to him.

But neither of us could fully commit to it. I don't know if it was because it had been too long since I had heard from God about his name, or the pressure that it had to be perfect, I kept doubting myself. And I was kind of testing Laxman about it. To the extent that I even confused him several times when he was firm with his decision all because of my indecisiveness.

We only had to come up with one name since we decided right from the start that we wouldn't be giving him a middle name. Even then, it was so difficult to decide on one name. Up until two weeks before the estimated due date, we were still thinking about it. Even when our families were asking us if we had chosen a name and offered some suggestions, our answer was that we would know when he was born. We didn't want any other suggestions or opinions. If it was from God, we would know it ourselves. We always said, "We will know what his name is the minute we see him in person." So, we reserved all our choices and kept it to ourselves.

Two days before 13th April (the day Levi was born), Laxman came running to me and suggested another name that was completely out of our own criteria. I was shocked! I didn't like it one single bit despite its meaning, and it definitely didn't suit us as a family or even the baby for that matter. The more I told Laxman I disliked the name, the more he tried to convince me. It was partially my fault; every time he referred to the baby as Levi, I would question him, asking if he was sure about it, making him go back to the drawing board. When he really did go back to the drawing board and came back with another name, I knew for a fact that it had to be Levi and nothing else.

If I am completely honest with myself, we both wanted to name him Levi from the very beginning, but we were looking for more reasons that it was his name. More like a direct voice from up above with thunder crashing and signs up with flashing lights saying Levi was his name, just like one of those "Santa, stop here!" sign boards during Christmas.

Well, obviously none of that happened. However, Laxman suggesting another name undoubtedly confirmed to me that Levi was his name. I wonder if he was testing me like I did to him?

When we left home on the morning of 13th April 2021 when my waters broke, we didn't even think of a name. The minute Levi was born that evening, he was given to me for a couple of minutes of skin-to-skin contact and then whisked away to be cleaned, checked and dressed up. I was being stitched while Laxman was with the midwives overlooking them. I was listening to their conversation while screaming through the gas and air tube that I was biting onto. One of the midwives asked Laxman if we had a name for him. Laxman answered without missing a beat or discussing with me, that he is Levi. In that very moment, I welled up and shed a tear. I had not cried the entire day throughout all the pain, pushing, tearing, or even panics, but the minute I heard Laxman name him Levi, he was confident. He just knew. Turns out, that's what I had been looking for all along. We both knew he was Levi, even before he was born, and even more so once we laid our eyes on him.

Later that evening, when Laxman texted our family and friends to announce the birth of our baby boy and his name, and we received nothing but awe-ness (I know it's not a word, but I don't know how else to describe their reactions) about his name, especially from my over-ambitious and over-achieving family who had so much expectation about the name.

So, what's the pride?

We are rather deep into this chapter, all I've spoken about is how Laxman and I decided not to do the screening test at twelve weeks, how the midwife described our baby as perfect from all the scans she'd done at twenty weeks, and how we ended up naming our son Levi. By now you may be wondering how on earth does any of this relate to pride.

When God first promised about the child, a son, and his name, I took it rather lightly. A year or two later, I would check in with God regularly to remind Him about the promise that He had given me, as if He needed that reminder to fulfil it. Three years later, I was holding God accountable for all my plight and the humiliation that I was facing. Four years later, I was plagued with doubt. I started questioning the promise and decided that I had made it all up, it was all in my mind and that it wasn't really from God at all like I had originally thought it was. I became bitter and refused to accept any sort of consolation from Laxman. I would retaliate and lash out towards anyone who asked me when they were going to hear "the good news" from me.

It was so difficult to stay focused on His promises during those five hazy years, that I resorted to living in denial of ever hearing it to begin with. I went through a turmoil of doubt and took everything seasoned with a mountain of salt. But six years down the road, here I am writing this chapter in the middle of the night while cradling my nine-month-old baby, who's peacefully sleeping in my arms after his night feed.

The promise was true. It was God. It was real. I really did hear God tell me about the generation. It was God who told me it was going to be a boy and it was definitely God who told me he will be called Levi. It wasn't my imagination. It wasn't just in my mind.

And do you know what else is better? That God fulfilled His promises. While the promise was from Him, it was only He who was able to fulfil it according to His perfect timing. Absolutely nothing I did in my own effort to help God fulfil His promise worked (or at least in my case).

Although the many long years in between did not reflect this, I am now able to look back and know for sure that it was God all along. The first voice, the first promise, the delays, the wait, everything was Him. I can be a bit thick sometimes that I need more signs and assurance than an ordinary person so that I can be sure I heard it right. For someone like me, who always needs double assurance, hearing from God once and then faced with silence for many years is completely unacceptable.

With all this realisation, I am proud and feel absolutely honoured that I heard Him the first time six years ago.

I just cannot say it enough that it really was God, and He spoke to me. I heard Him right the first time. To what do I owe such honour that God speaks to me?

Epilogue

Congratulations! You've made it to the last chapter of this book. *What a long-winded way of explaining God's promise and how He fulfilled it,* you must be thinking. Don't worry, I feel the same way too. It would have been far too easy to describe the last six years in one sentence.

I heard a promise from God, didn't believe it at first, started counting on it after some time, became frustrated when nothing happened, started doubting it and ended up denying it in my head. However, the story ended with the fulfilment of the promise.

Classic God-move, isn't it?

But that wouldn't have been real. If someone were to share with me their life-changing experiences in a sentence like above, it would trigger me to be even more furious that everything was so easy for everyone else but me. To me, it definitely sounds easy when said so briefly.

I wanted to keep it real for you and it's not real if you don't understand the details. It's so important to know the details because God is in the details. He cares about the details. Throughout all those years of struggling in my mind and flesh, trying to fight God and negotiate with Him, I was never alone. There were times when I refused to pray while Laxman prayed, because I didn't feel able to speak about anything else other than this one single thing that I got fed up with my own grumbling self.

It may seem as if I've been talking about myself and what I went through personally, but it's not really about me. Through every step of the way, God was there. He was there when there were delays at the fertility clinic appointments. He was there when my blood tests got lost multiple times. He was there when I was told the NHS wouldn't fund me. He was there when I found cheaper alternatives (*talk about being thick, I didn't get the hint at all that God was probably trying to say something to me through all these delays*). He was there when Laxman and I decided to delay alternative routes multiple time. He was there when He gave me the initial promise. He was also there when He told me we would only have a child once Laxman finished his PhD.

Did that last sentence catch you off guard? There was one more teeny tiny little detail that I haven't shared with you yet.

For a long time even after Levi was born, I believed that this was a very difficult journey because it took us such a long time to get to where we are. One fine day, the realisation suddenly dawned on me that it was only difficult because I made it difficult. Had I listened and taken to heart every detail that God gave me, it would have saved me from a lot of heartache that I put myself through because of my own doings.

You know how I explained about the promise that God gave me in 2015 and then there was silence for a good couple of years after that? It wasn't complete radio silence. Probably upon my insistence and pestering, God dropped a hint somewhere along the line that we would only have a child after Laxman completed his PhD. He was in his second year of the four-year programme when God told me this. Was I happy with this new hint? Nope! I was furious. I told God I couldn't sit around waiting for another two or three years. It's not like it was two or three months. How could I ever stop my impatient self from going into overdrive mode? This was around the end of 2017 when we were in the process of purchasing our house and had paused our fertility investigative journey for the time being.

I remember sharing this with Laxman, during one of our evening walks in the new neighbourhood, that God was only going to open the door for us once he'd finished his PhD. He was listening to me but did not respond. I contemplated repeating it, thinking he might not have heard it. But he did. He let out a faint acknowledgement. Man of few words.

So, that was that. We never spoke about it again, and I promptly forgot (I really did) about this new detail God had given me and carried on with the hustle and bustle of life, contemplating further surgeries, fighting with the NHS about the delays and more lost blood samples.

Laxman finished his write up by the end of 2019, and due to delays caused by the pandemic in early 2020, he had his viva booked for 15th July 2020 via Zoom. It was an all-day ordeal, but his external examiners confirmed to him at the end of the day that he had passed his PhD with only minor corrections. Three weeks later, on 5th August 2020, we found out we were pregnant using an expired pregnancy test. Only this time, it was for real and for good.

The teeny tiny detail that I had forgotten, the one where God said we would only have a child after Laxman completed his PhD, I still didn't remember it until we were much later into the pregnancy. It suddenly hit me like a ton of bricks. It didn't take us five years; it only took three weeks according to God's planning.

Have you ever heard that you must undergo a process in order to receive a promise? I have. Multiple times indeed, via sermons from so many different preachers. They always say that when God gives you a promise, it is accompanied by a process. The idea of it sounded acceptable when heard on TV or podcasts but didn't feel real until I endured it. I only wanted the promise and didn't want to experience the process. To be honest, I wasn't even aware of the process because I was so fixated on the promise.

Today, when Laxman and I look back at our journey and the process we underwent, I see how practical and thoughtful God has been. We were not financially stable to be able to provide for a baby like we are now, didn't have a good house that was safe and clean for a baby, Laxman wouldn't have been able to be as involved throughout the pregnancy as he was if he were still working on his PhD. I wouldn't have been ready to be a mother. More importantly, we wouldn't be as appreciative and aware of this blessing that we now call our son. These are only some of the things that I could think of. God has His timing and His reasons. There's no way we would have understood any of it if He had explained it to us back then.

During my virtual baby shower organised by my lovely E5 Church ladies, one of them pointed out to me that the number 5 means grace. I was given the promise in August 2015, and it was fulfilled in August 2020. That's five years! Oh, how gracious has God been. I surely needed that grace. Grace is God's unmerited favour as a result of God's love. There is absolutely no way I could have earned it or deserved it. I never thought I had a calling to be a mother. I never even thought that I was a very loving person with motherly qualities or instincts. But I love being Levi's mother.

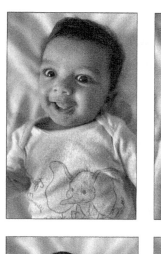
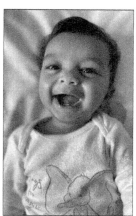
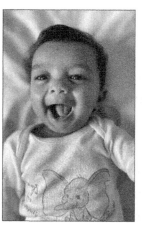
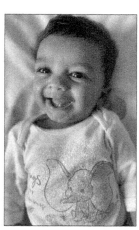
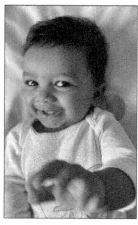

Amongst all the miracles God has done in my life to date, I don't feel like anything else can top this now, but I know my God. I know He has greater miracles in store for me, and for you.

The process looks very different for different people. In our case, God wanted us to be a lot more settled so that Levi could have complete undivided attention from his parents, and He had to work on my heart. Laxman had to finish his PhD, while I had to learn to trust God and be patient. Of course, I trust God and have faith in Him (despite questioning it at times). Have I now learnt to be patient? Sometimes, some questions are better left unanswered.

As months and years pass by, it's becoming more and more evident to me that this is not just my story. This is the story of many women out there. Your process and journey could be very different from mine, but the destination is the same: the promise. When there is a large gap between the promise and receiving it, doubt creeps in and throws everything off balance.

To all those who are on your journey of going through a process, if God has made a promise to you, hold on to it. Whether you are running, walking, limping or barely crawling through, keep doing it at any cost. It's such a cliché thing to say that when the going gets tough, the tough get going, but it's true. I could give you hundreds of verses from the Bible that say God will not leave you nor forsake you and why you shouldn't give up. But I just want to reassure you that He will fulfil His promises. It might not be in your time or to your expectation, but it will be done. Your breakthrough is coming.

If you believe in Jesus Christ, then you can be certain that "it's going to be OK" really means "it's going to be OK", even if it is not according to your plans and expectations.

Epilogue

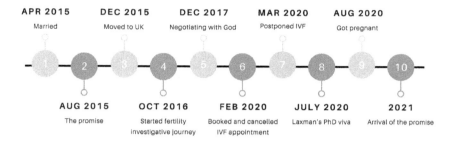

The Timeline

It's not about you, it's not about what you are or what you are not, it's not about what you have and haven't got. It's about God. It's always about him. God sees the end from the beginning, while we only see the beginning from the end.[9]

This song was a constant reminder of who God is and has sustained me through uncountable sleepless nights. I want to dedicate this song to you. You need it.

Way Maker[10]

You are here, moving in our midst
I worship You, I worship You
You are here, working in this place
I worship You, I worship You
You are here, moving in our midst
I worship You, I worship You
You are here, working in this place
I worship You, I worship You

You are Waymaker, miracle worker
Promise keeper, light in the darkness
My God, that is who You are
You are Waymaker, miracle worker
Promise keeper, light in the darkness
My God, that is who You are

You are here, touching every heart
I worship You, I worship You
You are here, healing every heart
I worship You, I worship You
You are here, turning lives around
I worship You, I worship You
You are here, mending every heart
I worship You, yeah, I worship You, Lord

You wipe away all tears,
You mend the broken heart
You're the answer to it all, Jesus
You wipe away all tears,
You mend the broken heart
You are the answer to it all, to it all, Jesus

To all the women out there who are still waiting for your bundle of joy, promises and dreams to be fulfilled, I kneel with you in prayer. May you receive peace like no other. Blessed shall be the fruit of your body, and the fruit of your ground, and the fruit of your animals, the increase of your cattle, and the young of your flock.[11]

It's going to be OK.

Endnotes

1. 1 Samuel 1:9-28.

2. Genesis 12:2.

3. Genesis 13:16.

4. Exodus 7 – 11.

5. WHO, 2021 https://www.who.int/health-topics/plague#tab=tab_1 (accessed February 2022).

6. Genesis 16.

7. Jackie Mize, *Supernatural Childbirth* (Harrison House, 1993).

8. "Famous For". Songwriter(s): Alexis Slifer, Chuck Butler, Krissy Nordhoff © Integrity's Praise! Music/BMI, Nordained Music/BMI (adm at IntegrityRights.com), Unknown.

9. Isaiah 46:10.

10. "Way Maker (Original Lyrics)". Songwriter(s): Osinachi Kalu Okoro Egbu © 2016 Integrity Music Europe (Adm. by CapitolCMGPublishing.com excl. UK & Europe, adm. by Integrity Music, part of the David C Cook family, songs@integritymusic.com)

11. Deuteronomy 28:4.